Fulfilled

Fulfilled

Let Go of Shame, Embrace Your Body,
and Eat the Food You Love

Alexandra MacKillop

BROADLEAF BOOKS
MINNEAPOLIS

Contents

Preface
vii

CHAPTER ONE
Our Deepest Need
Where Diet Culture Gets It Wrong
1

CHAPTER TWO
The Root of the Problem
Why Our Culture Is So Obsessed with Dieting
15

CHAPTER THREE
The Problem with Dieting
(and the Misleading Messages in the Media)
27

CHAPTER FOUR
Health at Every Size
You Don't Have to Be Thin to Be Healthy
43

CHAPTER FIVE
Eating with Freedom
God's Design for the Role of Food in Human Life
57

CHAPTER SIX

Making the Decision

The Most Important Step toward Intuitive Eating

71

CHAPTER SEVEN

Cultivating Awareness

Learning to Mindfully Listen to Your Body

91

CHAPTER EIGHT

Building a Foundation for Food Freedom

Focus on Adequacy, Variety, and Balance

113

CHAPTER NINE

Redeeming the Forbidden Fruit

A Systematic Approach to Breaking Food Rules

125

CHAPTER TEN

Guarding Your Heart

(against the Temptation to Diet)

137

CHAPTER ELEVEN

Final Thoughts

155

Appendix

161

Notes

171

Preface

I magine a life without dieting, without worrying about your weight, and without ever thinking about calories. Exercise is enjoyable, your clothes fit well, you eat your favorite foods on a regular basis, and you're at peace with the woman you see in the mirror.

Does that scenario sound unrealistic to you? Do you think it seems too good to be true to be able to eat whatever you're craving but stay in the same size clothes? Does it seem like a far-fetched daydream to be able to enjoy your favorite foods without worrying about what it will do to your waistline? I used to think so. At one point in my life, I wouldn't have believed it was possible to ever reach a place where I could go even ten minutes without worrying about nutrition labels, calorie counts, or the size and shape of my body. From age thirteen to age twenty, my life revolved around diet, exercise, and the number on the scale.

I started my first diet as a high school freshman because I thought it would help me with my athletic goals, but it quickly became much more than a performance-boosting tool. It took over my life, and I became completely obsessed with food. Cutting back on sweets turned into counting calories, worrying about workouts, and compulsively weighing myself—sometimes three or four times per day. I was fifteen when I was diagnosed with anorexia, significantly underweight but still convinced that the girl I saw in the mirror was too fat. Working with a dietitian and therapist helped me gain back the much-needed weight, but my mind was still consumed with thoughts about food and my body for years afterward. Even though I was "recovered" from a physical standpoint, I was far from free. I was a slave to food, exercise, and my bathroom scale. But unlike the early high school days when my size-zero jeans were falling off of me, my struggles as a young adult weren't so outwardly apparent.

By the time I started college, I had become a self-proclaimed health expert, spending hours every day rewriting recipes to be fat-free, sugar-free, and lower in calories. I scoured health blogs for information about superfoods, constantly researched the newest healthy diet practices, and watched hours upon hours of documentaries about food, exercise, health, and weight loss. But behind my facade of wellness, I was hiding a debilitating secret: my clean eating throughout the day was followed by binge eating at night—and I was more ashamed of that fact than I had ever been of anything else in my life. Even worse, I felt more distant from God than I did before I became a Christian. I was living in a cloud of darkness. Despite my every effort to the contrary, I couldn't contain myself around sweets and snacks, I couldn't lose weight, and I felt completely out of control. I thought I was doing everything right, but instead, my life was falling apart. I felt ashamed, like I was a complete failure because I couldn't figure out something as seemingly simple as eating. But for me, eating wasn't simple at all.

In those seven years, I memorized the calorie count of almost every food imaginable. I counted, measured, and calculated them so frequently that I can even recall most of them today—everything from carrots to all-purpose flour to Double Stuf Oreos. But although those calorie counts are still hidden away in the corners of my mind, I really couldn't tell you how many calories I eat in a day. I probably couldn't even recall what I ate for dinner last night. Because today, I don't think about food all that much anymore.

Nowadays, my life is characterized by food freedom—like the previously described non-diet scenario. After spending so many years obsessing over diet and exercise and truly suffering because of it, I finally decided that enough was enough. My life needed to change; otherwise, I wouldn't want to keep living it anymore. I'll share more about the details of that challenging transition later, but for now, I'll tell you this: working through my enslavement to food so that I could eat a cookie without panicking afterward was a slow and sometimes painful process. But it was 100 percent worth it, and it's exactly what I'll be walking you through in the pages of this book. In the coming chapters, we will explore the world of dieting from a completely new perspective, uncovering everything from the dangers of yo-yo eating patterns to the spiritual ramifications of poor body image, and even discuss the reason our culture is so obsessed with weight loss in the first place. Then I'll guide you through the process of restoring your own relationship with food and your body through a framework called intuitive eating so that you too can learn to let go of shame, embrace your body, and eat the food you love without feeling overwhelmed. I've taught countless women over the years to do exactly that, and my hope in writing this book is to help you as well.

A Little More about My Background . . .

My own healing process—true, holistic healing—began when I was in college. I was studying food science at the time, with plans to pursue medical school after graduation. But as I continued to repair my relationship with food and likewise grow in my faith, I started to feel drawn toward a profession where I could help others manage their health from a more holistic approach, taking more than just a patient's symptoms into account. I wanted to help others heal not only from infectious disease or broken bones but also from the epidemic of dieting and from a broken relationship with food, as I had done. I finally discovered functional medicine, a field where primary health care providers are trained to evaluate patients within the greater context of their lives, including everything from nutrition and exercise to stress levels, emotional well-being, and even spiritual practices. In addition to taking a closer look at their patients' lifestyles and histories, functional medicine physicians conduct detailed physical exams, run blood tests, order imaging, and more. As a provider in this field, I have the freedom (and time) to work with my patients more intensively to help them heal not only physically but also in every other dimension of their well-being.

Throughout my health care experience, the magnitude of the diet problem in our culture has become overwhelmingly apparent to me. Almost every woman I talk to, in a clinical setting or otherwise, can relate to the experience of food struggles, body shame, and frustrations related to fitness. Dieting is everywhere, and it destroys people's livelihoods. Not only do our food obsessions pose an enormous risk to our emotional and spiritual well-being, but they also wreak significant spiritual havoc on us. In dieting, we attempt to control what we ultimately cannot, and we lose sight of our true source of value and worth, which is Christ. Each of us is dearly loved by our creator, and his desire is for us to internalize and lean into that truth. God didn't place us on this earth just to count calories and follow an exercise plan; his desire is for us to thrive in light of his grace, kindness, and compassion—the things that truly give us worth and identity in this life. In my own struggles, I thought, like so many other women, that dieting would help me like my body more. But instead, it had the opposite effect—I became even more self-critical, and it made me forget just how loved I already was. It also made me physically sick.

The toll that my eating disorder took on my well-being completely negated any benefit that my diet initially might have provided. My extreme eating habits created significant physical health problems—a heart arrhythmia, fainting spells, and crippling stomach pain. This might sound surprising, but I wasn't even underweight when these symptoms emerged. On the outside, I looked healthy, but I was far from it: if I hadn't been able to heal when I did, I probably wouldn't be alive to write this book. I don't want anyone else to fall prey to diet demons—I've been there, and I know how awful it feels. Instead, I want to help as many women as possible heal their relationships with their bodies and learn to truly enjoy food and exercise, just as God intended for us.

As a Side Note . . .

In *Fulfilled*, I'll be talking a lot about the importance of rejecting food rules, eating treats, and embracing the areas of imperfection in our bodies. Initially, it might seem like I'm encouraging an attitude of flippancy toward health. I'm not, and here's why: food and nutrition influence our levels of physical wellness, and most individuals are well aware of this fact. But despite having this knowledge, millions of people still struggle to establish balanced, health-promoting eating patterns. There's a missing link between thoughts and behavior, and it is in our hearts. Until we confront the underlying beliefs and attitudes that influence our eating, we can't make headway in establishing good nutrition habits. While the processes required to conquer our food demons as presented in this book might not seem healthy at first, I promise that they ultimately lead down that road.

For example, overeating is a common struggle among women. In this book, I will explain why the best way to beat overeating and binge eating is to eat *more*, not *less*. See, it's our avoidance of chips, cookies, and other snacks that leads us to mentally disconnect and consequently overeat. At the end of the day, the problem is *dieting*, not food. Avoiding dessert doesn't necessarily prevent overeating or weight gain, and it often makes those problems worse. The other option is to stop avoiding our favorite foods and embrace them instead. The following chapters will explore this paradox and others in much greater detail. But I first want to preface the book with this: my message is pro-health. I believe that God wants us to care for our bodies, and therefore I want to encourage that message of self-care for all women, everywhere. While the means that I present for achieving the goal of health might be different from everything you've been told about nutrition throughout your entire life, I promise I'm not trying to trick you. The intuitive eating methods I'll share in these pages are backed by science, and I believe in them wholeheartedly. My own life is a testimony to the efficacy of exercising freedom in eating, and I hope the same for you. So if you're ready for a new food foundation that is built upon God's love for you instead of the false claims and shame of diet culture, read on!

CHAPTER ONE

Our Deepest Need

Where Diet Culture Gets It Wrong

I f you're reading this book, you probably have been on a diet at some point in your life or, at the very least, have tried to use food and exercise to change the size and shape of your body. You're not alone in this. Research shows that most people are dissatisfied with their appearances, and even girls as young as nine years old attempt to diet and lose weight. What most of us have come to realize, however, is that dieting isn't a very effective or lasting way to support well-being. Instead, it generally makes us feel awful, trapping us in a cycle of food preoccupation and body shame. It also pulls us further away from the very thing our hearts need most, which is to experience the all-encompassing, transformational, and wholly satisfying love of Christ. While dieting leaves us empty, God's love offers us fulfillment beyond measure.

Given the culture in which we live, feeling dissatisfied with our appearance is not only a common sentiment, but it's a completely understandable one too. Our culture makes us, as women, believe that our value and worth begin with our appearances. When the mirror doesn't reflect the photoshopped bodies plastered across our TV screens and Instagram feeds, dissatisfaction, frustration, and shame begin to bubble up in our hearts. Different diet companies then sell us their own branded solutions to our dissatisfaction, offering us weight-loss plans and exercise schedules designed to sculpt and chisel our bodies into the precise forms we desire. But when those diet and exercise plans fail to provide the results they promised, as they often do, all those negative feelings that led us to diet in the first place only intensify. In response, we move on to the next diet, and the next, and the next, until our dieting efforts completely consume our lives. Or, amid our exasperation, we give up on dieting and exercise completely, bring home a cart full of all the snacks our food rules previously forbade, and revel in our diet rebellion while bingeing on both Netflix and ice cream.

Most of us who have been in this situation end up blaming ourselves. But in reality, the diets failed us—not the other way around. As I will discuss throughout this book, there are countless reasons that diets don't work, but it's not because we lack willpower or because we're addicted to sugar. Rather, it's because the rationale behind dieting is fundamentally flawed. The reason for our poor self-image isn't that our bodies are too big; it's that they're too small to ever truly fulfill us. We've misdiagnosed our shame struggles as a physical problem when in reality they're spiritual.

The Wrong Diagnosis

Pause and think for a moment about the diet and fitness advertisements you see in grocery aisles, on billboards, and online. The arguments they use have quite a bit in common, don't they? The diet industry capitalizes on our body image struggles, telling us that the biggest problem in our lives is the inadequacy of our appearances. In turn, they offer us the latest diet as a one-size-fits-all solution. But this message gets it wrong in two key places: first, dieting doesn't help us feel better in our bodies, and second, weight loss isn't our deepest need in life. So when we struggle with feelings of guilt and shame about our appearances and set out to diet as an attempted solution, it's like taking the wrong prescription medication for our medical diagnosis. Not only do we not get the results we expect, but we put ourselves at enormous risk in the process.

Instead of enjoying our bodies more, we often feel worse about them as a result of dieting. Alongside that shame often comes a wide variety of other uncomfortable symptoms that range from fatigue and irritability to depression and self-loathing. In the next chapter, I'll uncover just how significant these problems are in terms of the breadth and depth of their effect on our physical, emotional, and spiritual health. But for now, let's focus on the end result, or lack thereof: diets don't deliver any of the benefits they promise, and frankly what most of us really need has far less to do with food and weight than what we give those things credit for. Instead, we need to turn our focus away from dieting, which drains us of energy, confidence, and satisfaction, and toward Christ, who truly fulfills us.

For most of us, dieting has less to do with our bodies and more to do with the pressures we put on ourselves. In moments of low confidence, stress, or life changes, our discomfort drives us to take action—someway, somehow. But instead of looking to the source of those uncomfortable feelings, we turn inward—or rather, outward toward our bodies. We start dieting in the hope that changing the number on the scale will change the way we feel about ourselves. Think about the reasons women typically cite for wanting to lose weight: bouncing back after having a baby, getting ready for bikini season, feeling more confident, fitting into old jeans, preparing for a wedding, and so on. Although these are understandable reasons for dieting given the cultural pressures we face, whittling down a few extra pounds doesn't cure the underlying sense of dissatisfaction, anxiety, or low self-esteem that leads us to desire weight loss in the first place. After the number on the scale changes, we are still ourselves. We are still the same moms, sisters, wives, friends, and daughters; the same doctors, teachers, artists, and homemakers; the same quirky, unique, and imperfect women we were at the beginning. But most importantly, we are still loved by God.

Our True Identities

The way God views us doesn't match up with the way that many of us view ourselves. God doesn't look down from heaven and say, "Hmm, she would be prettier if she just lost a few pounds" or "She'd be a much better wife and mom if she cut calories a bit." No, in the Bible, we read that we are *fearfully and wonderfully made* and *dearly loved*. What's more, God spoke those truths over us before we were even born. In the beginning, the earth was empty and dark. But in his wisdom and love, God willingly chose to create something from nothing, the visible from the invisible, sons and daughters in his very own image. When he was finished, he called his creation "very good" (Genesis 1:31). Friends, God didn't make a mistake when he made your bodies. When he designed you, he acted intentionally and with great care, breathing life into your lungs with purpose and promise. Even today, when he beholds the human form, he delights in his own artistry, each of us specially made with love, by love, to be loved. When we adopt a condemning attitude toward our bodies on the basis of appearance, we create distance between ourselves and God, defying his proclamation that we were made beautiful by him. Instead of reflecting his kindness, grace, and gentleness, dieting leads us to criticize and judge his creation. What we need most in life isn't to lose twenty pounds. Doing so won't make our lives better, it won't make us more valuable, and it won't fulfill our hearts. No, our deepest need is to understand the full weight of the truth that God loves us with an incomprehensible love not because of how we look but because of who we are: his own.

In today's diet-obsessed culture, the idea of a diet-free life is entirely radical and even almost risqué. In fact, some might argue that allowing our bodies to self-regulate eating and exercise behavior would be irresponsible. (This is the driving force behind pretty much every formal diet plan.) After all, wouldn't permitting people to eat whenever they're hungry be essentially allowing them to self-destruct? Aren't humans inherently prone to gluttony and sloth? Once again, we can look to the

Bible for truth. In the beginning, food matters were plain and simple: "The Lord God took the man and put him in the Garden of Eden to work it and take care of it. And the Lord God commanded the man, 'You are free to eat from any tree in the garden'" (Genesis 2:15–16). When God created the first man and woman, he didn't also give them diet plans. Rather, he created them with the ability to choose when, where, and how much to eat. He provided them with everything they needed to enjoy a life free and at peace with food, with God, and with their own bodies. We read in Genesis 2:25 that even though Adam and Eve were naked and exposed, they felt no shame—a truth completely contrary to the messages of diet culture. Instead of helping us embrace the uniquely beautiful bodies that God created for each of us, dieting drives us toward guilt, fear, and isolation.

Dieting Begets Shame

Food is a unique part of life in that we need to think about it in order to survive. It demands our attention three times a day, like clockwork. Anytime we think about something so much, we face the temptation to get carried away. At least, that was my experience. As a young woman, I thought that to perform well in sports, support my health, and maintain a body shape and size I was comfortable with, I needed to be careful about what and how much I was eating. During my adolescent years, health and nutrition were hot topics in the media, and I took everything I read and heard very seriously. I created strict rules for myself about the types and amounts of food I'd allow myself to eat, and I didn't deviate much from them for the first few months of dieting. Everything was under control—until it wasn't anymore.

With time, my eating habits became more and more restrictive, and I kept limiting what I ate long after the state competitions came and went. I was furious when my mom brought me to the doctor and lamented my restrictive habits. I became even more frustrated when I started seeing a nutritionist who prescribed a meal plan very different from my self-imposed one, and I was horrified when my parents started enforcing it at home. (I didn't think I really had a problem, so I didn't expect my parents to take it that seriously.) I resisted for a while but finally surrendered after my well-intentioned but concerned parents threatened to take me off my cross-country team, ground me from my phone, and keep me from driving. It's a little awkward to think back on the things that motivated me at that time, but I share them because they illustrate a key point: I wasn't ready to give up my food rules. I changed my habits reluctantly. I ate the foods I didn't want to eat and gained the weight I didn't want to gain, but it only lasted for a little while.

It wasn't long before life began to feel overwhelming, as it tends to, and I returned to the only coping mechanism I knew: food rules. Although I didn't understand how or why it was happening, I started to see a big difference in my body's reaction to my restrictions—it fought back. I skipped meals and avoided necessary nutrients like carbohydrates and fat throughout the day, but I soon became overwhelmed by urges to eat those types of foods in the evening. When I started bingeing, I was terrified. Why couldn't I control myself around the tempting cookies and jars of peanut butter like I once could? What had happened to my self-control? I didn't know what was wrong with me. I was afraid I was broken. But I didn't realize that the very opposite was true. My body was behaving the way it was designed to behave in times of starvation. I needed food, and biology was taking over despite my mental efforts to the contrary. I was losing in the battle against myself.

The inner turmoil I experienced at that time is what I now refer to as food shame, a common side effect of dieting. Food shame results when we begin viewing ourselves as unworthy, inadequate, or otherwise less-than because of our failure to comply with the food rules we impose on ourselves. Where God tells us we are loved regardless of what, when, or how much we eat, food shame tells us that we are unworthy if we fail to live up to our eating or exercise standards. Food shame tells us that we're out of control, that we lack willpower, and that we are failures. Sometimes these shame-driven self-narratives even stretch out into other areas of our identities, as if a "sweet tooth" is akin to a character flaw. Food shame feeds us the lie that what we eat defines who we are.

Body shame is no different. This phenomenon emerges from the disconnect between what we look like and what we think we need to look like in order to deserve love, esteem, or value. Body shame tells us that outward appearance trumps all and that there's something wrong with us if we don't look a certain way. Just as I felt broken and ashamed because I couldn't maintain my food rules, I was horrified by the changes taking place in my body because of my binges. I desired to be thin above all else, and nothing in my life seemed to matter as much as the scale did. But learning the truth eventually set me free. Throughout the Bible, we read that we can't earn value and significance in God's eyes no matter how hard we try, whether by what we eat or what we look like. Instead, he offers his love to us as a free gift, inviting us to then go and share that love with others.

Understanding and internalizing my identity in Christ was fundamental to my recovery. For years, I tried to get a handle on my eating disorder by following the strict rules I'd made for myself. But what held me back was my mistaken belief that I needed to use my mind to override my body's signals to maintain my weight and that I needed to keep my weight in check to be valuable. Finally, by God's grace, I learned that my body was designed to self-regulate. God knew what he was doing when he created us and placed us on this earth. He really meant it when he said we didn't need to be afraid, whether in terms of our body sizes, the food we eat, or anything else in life. His design was perfect the first time, and we can consequently trust the bodies he gave us. We can trust our bodies' hunger signals, we can trust their promptings for rest, and we can trust that when the scale fluctuates, it's normal, healthy, and good. Trusting this internal process of self-regulation is called intuitive eating.

Eating with Freedom

In the 1990s, dietitians Evelyn Tribole and Elyse Resch recognized that dieting wasn't helping their patients lose weight or improve their health. Furthermore, it wasn't equipping them to live happier or more vibrant lives; their dieting actually caused them suffering! On the other hand, they noticed that people who were very closely attuned to their body cues were able to effortlessly maintain their body weight within a healthy range (which is different for each and every body). Tribole and Resch referred to these individuals as *intuitive* eaters, meaning they allowed their own intuition and attunement to their bodies to determine what, when, and how much they ate. They also noticed that these intuitive eaters incidentally had the healthiest physiologic wellness markers, such as blood pressure and cholesterol levels. Intuitive eaters, curiously, paid less attention to the nutrition labels of the foods they were eating and more attention to their internal sense of hunger and fullness, satisfaction, and emotional needs. Inspired by these findings, Tribole and Resch stopped recommending weight-loss diets to their patients and instead dedicated their efforts toward helping them become intuitive eaters. Though paradoxical, it was the truth: the less their patients concerned themselves with nutrition, the healthier they became.

Intuitive eating refers to an approach to food in which there are no good or bad foods, no right or wrong mealtimes, and neither desserts, nor snacks, nor rich ingredients are off-limits. It altogether removes food rules and instead puts the power back into the hands of you, the eater, to feed yourself whenever you are hungry with whichever foods you so choose. Through this exercise of freedom, you are then able to explore how you feel when you eat any given type of food and then use that knowledge to inform your food choices going forward. What this looks like in practice is eating a donut for breakfast if that's what sounds good but at the same time recognizing that the donut might not provide lasting energy. Eating with freedom allows you to enjoy sweets, even first thing in the morning, but empowers you to make the choice to include eggs or yogurt for protein too. Likewise, it enables you to choose a light salad for lunch fueled by the knowledge that a heavier meal might make you too drowsy to endure your afternoon work meeting. Intuitive eating permits you to enjoy an abundance of both delicious and nutritious food as a means of self-care inspired by God's love and care for you.

In my initial appointments with patients, I'll often ask them a follow-up question after they explain their current eating and exercise patterns: "Are you doing this because you love your body or because you don't?" More often than not, they answer with the second option. See, diet and fitness plans don't come from a place of acceptance and satisfaction with our bodies as they are. They come from a place of criticism. We don't like how we look, so we start taking steps to change our appearances: food rules, running schedules, weekly weigh-ins. Because we live in a society that scrutinizes every part of the human form, it's difficult to feel good in our own skin even when we are perfectly healthy. So we diet. Intuitive eating, on the other hand, is all about letting ourselves be. Unlike diets, intuitive eating focuses on responding to what our bodies are telling us rather than what the world is telling us. It likewise inspires us to make food choices that honor God's design rather than the designs of Photoshop editors. When we eat intuitively, we're set free from the suffering and struggles that come with trying to micromanage our weight. Diets drain our energy and joy, but choosing to honor our internal body signals through intuitive eating allows us to fill our hearts and minds with more than just the physical parts of ourselves. In fact, it allows us to be filled—and fulfilled—by the very thing we were designed for: God's love.

Food Freedom and Health

On my blog, where I write more about intuitive eating and food freedom, I often receive reader questions about the limitations of intuitive eating, such as situations when eating a brownie might not be the best choice. Likewise, you might now be thinking that intuitive eating sounds great but are at the same time wondering about the health implications. After all, aren't snack foods the reason for America's obesity epidemic? Don't we need to be stricter about our diets rather than more relaxed? Don't worry, we'll get there. This topic will be covered in much more detail in chapter 4. But for now, the most important thing to keep in mind is that most people aren't currently eating intuitively. There's a big difference between honoring a craving and mindlessly finishing off a bag of potato chips, and this book will help you learn about that difference in detail. It's mindless overconsumption that causes problems, not conscientiously responding to our internal signals. Intuitive eating equips us with the skills we need in order to allow our bodies to self-regulate—a process that God designed in the very beginning but that dieting prevents.

When God created us, he chose to include the need for us to eat regularly, but he also equipped us with a sufficient level of natural intuition to inform our food choices. Yes, our bodies really can tell us when to put down the ice cream and pick up a carrot stick. They also can tell us when to head outside for a hike and when to stay in and rest. We just need to learn to listen. I'll admit that I had my concerns about trusting my body at first too. I was afraid that my cravings would never end and that I'd eat myself to death. But that didn't happen, and I'm physically healthier nowadays while eating dessert every night than I was when I avoided it like the plague. My mind is also much more at ease, as I also don't regularly weigh myself anymore or fantasize over a smaller pants size. Best of all, eating my favorite foods no longer sends me into a spiral of guilt, shame, and self-condemnation. As an intuitive, free eater, I know that obsessing over every morsel of food that I put into my mouth poses a far greater health risk than eating a brownie ever could.

For some, my excellent physical health compared to the frequency with which I eat dessert might not make sense. In fact, I've received numerous unsolicited comments about my apparent "fast metabolism," or I've been asked about my diet and exercise habits because my physique is seemingly desirable. Because I am a functional medicine physician, these folks expect me to share some sort of strict eating plan and are often shocked when I don't. I almost laugh when I think back to my college years, when I was a self-proclaimed "clean eater" but weighed twenty pounds more than I do now, suffered from high cholesterol (which developed due to my binge eating), felt constantly fatigued, and was overridden with food-related fears and anxiety. My mind was so consumed with thoughts about eating and exercise that I could focus on little else. My schoolwork suffered, my relationships suffered, and I felt so dark and distant from God that I questioned my faith. Once I turned away from dieting and instead cultivated an attitude of freedom in my eating, I finally became healthy—physically, emotionally, and most importantly, spiritually. This is a far cry from the assumptions that outsiders make about my lifestyle based on my appearance. But the assumptions are understandable given what we are taught about the relationship between body weight, food, and eating habits.

Sometimes when I encourage my patients to eat dessert, take rest days, or honor cravings, they worry that I hold a flippant attitude toward nutrition. This isn't true at all—I love nutrition and health, and I take them so seriously that I've focused my entire career on them. However, I also understand from both personal and professional experience that French fries don't hold the power of life and death. I've ultimately come to realize that the minutiae of nutrition are a lot less important to our health than our attitudes toward food. In some ways, what we eat doesn't really matter. Even throughout my years of education, I haven't been convinced that a "perfect human diet" exists, and I most certainly don't believe that food is the be-all and end-all. In fact, scientific research hasn't been able to find a universally accepted "ideal diet" either. Rather, current findings suggest that genetics and happenstance are far more influential on human health and disease than the composition of one's diet. Of course, balanced eating habits are very important in self-care, and it's wise to pay some attention to the food we consume. But dietary power is limited, and focusing too much on food or body weight is detrimental to our overall health. Toward the end of the book, I will discuss the ways we can reasonably exercise wisdom in terms of nutritional quality. However, I feel most women today are lacking not in their mental strength or scientific knowledge but in their ability to exercise *freedom* in their eating.

When I finally began to heal from my struggles with food, I was at a physically healthy weight but still very unwell emotionally and spiritually. It wasn't until I turned away from my false beliefs about food and instead embraced a paradigm characterized by freedom that I finally experienced the joy God intended for us in eating. For me, this meant giving up my pursuit of a "perfectly healthy" diet and intentionally choosing foods I was afraid of—things like desserts, snacks, and high-calorie restaurant meals. While this process seemed unbalanced in the beginning, I eventually started craving those "healthier" foods again and came to enjoy cookies and kale equally. By realizing that I had permission under God to enjoy sweets and treats, I was able to break free from my binge compulsions and instead eat intuitively, according to the signals my body was giving me about which foods to choose, how much to eat, and when.

My intent is not to convince you to not care about nutrition or not give thought to your body or to suggest that all diets are inherently bad. Rather, it is the opposite—to encourage you to care for your body *more* and to do it *better*. Through this book, I hope to show you that we don't need to fear food or resist natural changes in our physiques. As individuals who are beautifully created by God, we have the freedom to embrace our physical selves, enjoy the gift of pleasure in eating, and do both without fear of repercussions. God made us with the need to eat, and he also provided us with a way to meet that need that isn't nearly as difficult as the dieting industry has made it out to be. Our bodies are the means of spreading God's love in the world—they are holy vessels. Of course we should love and honor them! Therefore, this book will serve as a guide for cultivating a relationship with food and your body that honors God, reflecting his love to ourselves and others. Throughout the process, we must keep in mind that changing our approach to food is not as simple as flipping a switch. But with hard work, we can actively take steps to restore our relationships with both food and our bodies, reconciling our eating habits with God. Those who are in Christ are promised redemption in every area, so I promise you that if you share your food struggles with God, you will be met with abounding love and grace.

CHAPTER TWO

The Root of the Problem

Why Our Culture Is So Obsessed with Dieting

Intuitive, free eating is not the norm in our culture. Dieters far outnumber nondieters, and those who have never fallen prey to the temptation of food rules are few and far between. People don't need to have diagnosed eating disorders to struggle in their relationships with food. Somewhere on the spectrum between intuitive eaters and those with anorexia, binge eating disorder, and the like, we find a phenomenon called disordered eating. Unlike overt self-imposed starvation or purging behaviors, disordered eating is sneakier and subtler. It shows up in unusual but culturally acceptable ways, like skipping meals, eating out of boredom, cutting out food groups, or counting calories. Stated bluntly, dieting is disordered eating. While intuitive eaters mindfully honor hunger and fullness cues with the foods their bodies crave, dieters impose external rules on what, when, or how much they eat. But regardless of the name we give something—whether *dieting* or *disordered eating* or *eating disorder*—the dysfunction comes from the same place. When our needs aren't being met, when we're struggling with our sense of self, or when life feels out of control, we cling to whatever is closest to us that seems to fill that void. On an individual level, turning to food in those moments makes sense because diet behavior is all around us. Our diet education starts young, and when we grow up in a society that collectively suffers from disordered eating, it only makes sense that we will respond in kind.

Of course, we all have unique life experiences that affect our relationships with food, and it would be unfair to make generalizations about them by boiling our struggles down to "monkey see, monkey do." But the generalization *can* be made that we collectively look to dieting in an attempt to fix our problems because that's what we're taught to do. Dieting is modeled to us and advertised to us, and after a long pattern of participating in it ourselves, it becomes deeply ingrained within us. When dieting is the cultural norm, *not* dieting is wildly countercultural—and doing the countercultural thing is never easy. Despite the fact that swimming against the current is extremely difficult, resisting cultural diet norms is worth every bit of effort. Here's why: giving up dieting allows us to focus more on that which truly meets our needs, satisfies our desires, and empowers us toward a life of freedom. But in order to receive that satisfaction and freedom, we need to understand why we started dieting in the first place.

Dieting for Beauty

When I was in elementary school, my family visited the Museum of Science and Industry in downtown Chicago. One of the exhibits that most struck me as a young girl was a film discussing aesthetic traditions in different cultures throughout the ancient world. These included practices like chemical skin bleaching and foot binding in China, double-eyelid surgery in Japan and Korea, neck elongation in Myanmar, and lip plates in Ethiopian tribes. Many of these traditions created extreme disfigurations of the human form and would be considered horrifyingly abusive today. For example, neck elongation in Myanmar involves wrapping brass coils around the necks of young girls, gradually increasing the number of coils with age. The force of the coils depresses the collarbones into the rib cage, giving the appearance of a long neck. Although the vertebral column isn't actually lengthened, the force of the coils weakens the girls' neck muscles to the point where adult women cannot hold up their heads without the coils. The lip-plating procedure in teenage Ethiopian girls involves inserting plates of progressively larger diameter into a hole made in their lower lips. The plates are so large and impede the mouth so much that women often need to have some of their teeth removed! While these practices may seem unnatural and harmful, in their cultures, they signify beauty. Could the same be said about our own cultural practices?

In general, we understand that the stick-thin, supermodel appearance we see in magazines and on billboards is an unhealthy, unattainable standard. Although most of us may not expect to ever achieve the six-foot-tall, size-zero look, we manipulate our diets in hopes of inching just a little bit closer to that ideal. Unfortunately, chasing after these beauty standards paradoxically creates the opposite effect of our desired self-esteem improvement. Author Lisa Endlich Heffernan discussed this idea in a recent *Forbes* article: "Our relentless focus on our appearance and our inevitable failure to attain the standards of beauty we see around us erodes confidence, increases self-doubt, and consumes our energies."[1] Dietitians Evelyn Tribole and Elyse Resch likewise note in their book *Intuitive Eating* that "dieting is correlated with feelings of failure, lowered self-esteem, and social anxiety."[2] They also note the degree to which dieting and weight specifically tie into feelings of worthiness, citing research showing that many obese individuals believe that they could not have become obese unless they possessed some sort of "fundamental character deficit."[3] As a culture, we internalize outward criticism as inward flaws, forgetting our worth in the eyes of God.

It also doesn't help when we see everyday women perfectly posed, propped up, and photoshopped to appear as slim as possible in their Instagram feeds. Social media pages with thousands of followers typically are owned by naturally slim women and present a carefully curated thin ideal that seems to (but does not actually) reflect what the average adult woman can and should be. For an influencer, presenting an image that more closely matches the cultural beauty ideals means she will gain more attention on her posts. People literally *like* when they see thin women. Sometimes, this attention even translates into a monetary reward for those who make the posts. Although most of us don't earn money off our looks, we still earn esteem for our beautification efforts. I know in my own use of social media, my pictures are much more likely to receive positive feedback when my hair is curled, my makeup is done, and I'm wearing something other than my pajamas.

The more we see beauty as valuable in our communities—a phenomenon evidenced by social media influencer culture—the more easily we forget where our true value lies. While having a thin frame or a lean physique as a woman certainly isn't an inherently bad thing, God does not give us the desire to change our bodies to look like those of other women; our diet-obsessed culture does. The Bible tells us that we each are fearfully and wonderfully made (Psalm 139:14). This truth applies to every woman, everywhere, in every context. Whether tall or short, thick or thin, God names us "beloved." The idea that we need to look different to be loved and valued is a lie; God loves each of us, and he expressed this love in the unique ways he created each and every one of our bodies.

I remember a conversation with a Christian mentor in college during which she shared the struggle she and her husband were undergoing with their daughter, who was dying of complications from a rare genetic disease. She was near tears as she spoke, and I could see the despair in her face. But I knew she was clinging to the hope that what she was saying was true: "I have to believe that God created Katie purposefully—that he knew what he was doing when he knit her together as a tiny baby, when he gave her lungs that didn't work properly, but breathed life into them anyway. I have to believe that when he made her little body, he wasn't wrong, and he isn't wrong now as he is calling her back home." It was a heartbreaking and terrifying conversation, coming to terms with the brevity and fragility of life. In witnessing death, we are reminded of the utter lack of control we have over our bodies.

The truth is, each of our bodies will fail us eventually. For Katie, it happened in a significant way at a very early age. But I think we all can agree that Katie's disease didn't mean that she was any less loved by God. Her mother was correct: God wasn't wrong when he made her body, and he wouldn't have cared for her any more deeply if she had a different one. While for most of us, our body woes don't stem from terminal illnesses, the same holds true: God created each of us uniquely and loves us equally. He would not love us differently if we looked a different way or if we were to change our bodies' shapes and sizes. In other words, God will not love us more if we lose the baby weight, tone up, or slim down to finally fit into that pair of jeans. He loves us beyond what we can imagine just as we are, and it is up to each of us to choose to believe in that love.

Living in the culture that we do, a preoccupation with external beauty is perfectly understandable. People notice women who represent the present culture's beauty ideals. They get attention that other women don't. They are revered, praised, and painted on magazine covers. But outward appearance doesn't change God's love for us. If anything, focusing so much on appearance poses a distraction from *knowing* God's love for us and living fully in the freedom of our identity as his children—no dieting necessary. The more praise and affirmation we receive for weight loss and the more we see thin women on diet magazines, the more we believe that dieting brings us beauty and that beauty will satisfy our every desire. But instead, it will just continue to disappoint, robbing us of knowing the true value and beauty of our bodies, just as they are.

Dieting for Belonging

The pursuit of beauty is just one of the reasons women turn to diets. But diet culture also shows up in other areas of daily life, sometimes in unexpected ways. A few years ago, I participated in a seminar that was followed by a Chipotle-sponsored luncheon. As I made my way through the food line, a woman whom I'd never met turned to me and said, "You know, I've been doing intermittent fasting, and I've already lost ten pounds. I know this looks like a lot of food, but it'll be my only meal today." That was all she said, and then she walked away. Confused and taken aback, I just stared after her, wondering why in the world she chose to tell me that. I didn't even know her! *Did I do or say something that made her feel uncomfortable?* As far as I was aware, I'd been minding my own burrito.

After that incident, I found myself noticing similar diet talk among the women in my life. Whether they were living in large bodies or small ones, it seemed like ladies of all shapes and sizes constantly either commiserated over their food and fitness initiatives or offered unsolicited explanations as to why they were eating dessert. A few months after the incident with the woman at the Chipotle table, I came to the realization that her behavior had more to do with me than I'd realized. Or rather, it was a response to many of the other women, like me, who were in the room. If you're surrounded by a crowd of people who weigh less than you do in a cultural moment where thinness is praised, having a larger body is extremely isolating. Add that to the fact that the room was filled with health care providers sitting down to share a meal together, I can only imagine how judged she must have felt. I've also been the recipient of unsolicited comments about the amount of food on my plate, my choice to eat dessert, or my liberal application of butter, and even though I'm completely confident in my food choices, such comments still make my face flush. My favorite of all was a colleague who eyed the Goldfish crackers on my plate and said, "Just so you know, I'm not judging how many processed carbs you're eating right now. Don't worry, I ate some pasta last week. We all do it sometimes." I spent the rest of the afternoon fantasizing about all the sassy retorts I wished I'd given him instead of blushing and turning away.

When we feel ashamed of our bodies, we face enormous pressure to try to change them. If we can't change how we look, we make the effort to at least give the appearance of making choices that others would approve. For example, many women feel ashamed of their body weight, fearing judgment from others not only for how they look but for the food choices they make, as though the size and shape of their bodies are completely dependent on their diets. To compensate for this, they strive to present themselves as health advocates, hoping to earn a pardon for their present physique by proving that they're at least attempting to change. They share health-related articles on social media, cook "clean" recipes, and swap diet ideas with friends. The fear of being judged for their weight strongly motivates them to pursue "healthy eating" and other diet-related behaviors even if they aren't actually able to lose weight. By taking on the identity of dieters, they hope to gain the acceptance from their communities that their bodies couldn't earn them through thinness.

In the same way, many women feel that they need to put parts of their lives on hold until their bodies look a certain way. I used to refuse to wear a bathing suit at the beach or even swim at all because I felt I didn't look "fit enough." My preoccupation with my body led to my belief that I was unworthy of enjoying life. Instead, I sat on a towel, fully clothed, while my friends or family swam. Some of my patients have shared similar experiences with me, explaining that they put extra pressure on themselves to look a certain way before they feel they can participate in important life events. Whether by losing weight or toning up, they feel that others will respect them more and that they'll be more worthy of certain experiences or occasions if they change their bodies.

As women, we are encouraged to start new diets centered on almost every season of life. From summer "bikini-ready" initiatives, to weddings, to pregnancy, instead of encouraging us to embrace our present bodies, our culture places emphasis on changing them, specifically through dieting. But whether we succeed in our dieting goals or not, we end up spending weeks or months consumed with the pursuit of crafting an appearance of doing the "right thing" with food. But what so many of us fail to realize in these moments is that our value and worthiness in the eyes of God—or even in the eyes of our loved ones—are not dependent on what we eat, how much we exercise, or our respective levels of body fat. God's love for us is rooted in grace, mercy, and kindness and is in no way dependent on what we look like. He loves us because of *who we are*, not because of what we do, and certainly not because of what we do or don't eat for dinner. Believing otherwise allows a lie to distract us from the life of abundance that God offers us instead.

Dieting as a Religion

Another reason we are drawn to diets is that they carry an almost religious appeal. One of the most interesting food trends, in my opinion, has been the push to go gluten-free. While it's true that the consumption of high-carbohydrate, highly processed, gluten-containing grain products is an important consideration in chronic disease,[4] there is little evidence to show that naturally occurring levels of gluten *alone* cause these conditions (the obvious exceptions are autoimmunity and allergies). But as Alan Levinovitz describes in his book *The Gluten Lie*, the concept of avoiding certain foods for health benefits isn't new. Ancient Chinese monks once believed that the high-grain Chinese diet "rotted and befouled" the organs, leading to premature death.[5] Their philosophy became wildly popular, at least until bandwagon followers fell off and were ostracized, a process akin to excommunication from the modern church. Levinovitz recognizes a parallel between diet-specific groups and certain faith practices. Unequivocally, food beliefs and followings can become almost cult-like and religious: people devote time, energy, and resources to serving a food god, even forming community groups in weekly devotion. (Think Weight Watchers meetings, keto support groups, and vegan activism clubs.) Gathering together around the *avoidance* of certain foods creates community, identity, and a sense of acceptance that would be otherwise unavailable without dieting. The sense of morality we attach to food also feeds into the strikingly religious qualities of dieting. I'm not talking about concern for animal welfare or environmental consciousness but rather the guilt and shame that so often result from deviating from a set of food rules. These food rules come to be seen as spiritual laws (do not eat, do not drink, do not touch), and violation often leads to self-inflicted punishment. Take cookies, for example: the penance for a sinfully delicious dessert is a two-mile run, five hundred sit-ups, or a forty-five-minute gym session.

Purging behaviors like this are a hallmark sign of eating disorders, yet we normalize these actions in our society. Whenever we break the food rules we make for ourselves or our reflections in the mirror don't match up with what we'd prefer, we take drastic measures. We utilize special diets, detoxes, and the recently popular thirty-day "resets" specific to meat eaters, postpartum women, the holiday season, and nearly every other experience of life. But at the end of the day, we don't need to detox or reset anything to be loved by God. We already are. (Yes, you—right where you are, right now.) Nothing can separate us from that truth, no matter our life experiences, the food we eat, how much or little we exercise, or what we see in the mirror. Whether we detox or not, we are worthy of love and belonging.

Dieting for Control

Restricting and monitoring our diets also appeals to us because doing so offers us the illusion of control. My struggles with food and exercise started at a tumultuous time in my life. I'd just started high school, which probably says enough on its own. But in addition to the pressures I was facing in sports and academics, my sister had just moved to college, some of my close friends had transferred schools, and many of the students in my classes had attended different middle schools than I had, so I hardly knew anyone. I felt extremely isolated. Just when I'd started to feel like things were settling down; life would throw another plot twist at me. Focusing on food and fitness came as a very welcome comfort, something I actually could control. No matter what happened at school that day, I knew that one tablespoon of peanut butter would always have the same number of fat grams and that running a mile would always burn the same number of calories. It was safe and predictable, and I clung to it like a life preserver. But it was all an illusion.

Attempting to radically control our lives through dieting almost always backfires. In 1997, Dr. Steven Bratman began to notice that the extreme degree of dietary preoccupation and restriction of some people paradoxically created deleterious health consequences.[6] Social isolation, anxiety, and loss of the natural and intuitive ability to eat were only a few of the trends he noticed, and some were as severe as fatal malnutrition. He termed the condition *orthorexia nervosa*, which translates from Greek to mean "correct diet." Essentially, sufferers were so concerned with the health benefits of food that they were taking extreme measures in micromanaging nutrition. Today, the condition has come to affect so many individuals that it is a widely accepted term in modern medicine. Patterns exhibited by orthorexics include compulsive behavior and mental preoccupation with healthful diets, pervasive anxiety, and shame resulting from violating self-imposed dietary rules, along with increasing frequency and severity of detoxification measures. While orthorexics are not necessarily concerned with weight loss, they often see it as a sign of success. Truly, orthorexia's consequences present an ironic dichotomy for someone so painstakingly devoted to healthy eating.

Even outside the confines of an orthorexia diagnosis, many of us gravitate toward prescriptive or prohibitive diet plans because they give us a sense of security and safety. Every day, we face thousands of food-related decisions, in addition to the countless other choices we need to make throughout our daily lives. This ceaseless decision-making is stressful, so it's completely understandable that creating rules for ourselves about food or exercise brings us comfort. We're also faced with countless unknowns in our lives and things outside of our control. When it comes to health especially, the many unknowns are rather unnerving, so we tend to prefer anything that presumes to offer a solution over continuing to stumble through the darkness. Guidelines and limitations make us feel like we are the ones in control.

But that "feeling" of control is just that—a feeling. At the end of the day, we have very little control over our lives. Accidents happen all the time. Whether it's a job loss, a tragic fire, the death of a loved one, or an unforeseen diagnosis, the circumstances of tomorrow are completely outside the realm of our jurisdiction. Control is just one of the false promises of dieting. Obsessing over food and exercise doesn't make us more beautiful either. It doesn't create meaningful relationships for us, because the sense of collective belonging it gives is just an illusion. We need to connect with others, and with God, on a much deeper level than a watered-down conversation about food and exercise. Ultimately, dieting sets us up only to be let down because it can't follow through on its promises. Instead, it leaves us with problems far bigger than it ever offered to solve.

CHAPTER THREE

The Problem with Dieting
(and the Misleading Messages in the Media)

When I initially started recovery for my eating disorder, my treatment team addressed the physical health risks, such as my low weight, but I continued to struggle in my heart and mind. I started eating more regular meals and exercising less, but the dissatisfaction with my body remained. In fact, it actually worsened. Instead of worrying about whether I had lost enough weight, I started despising myself for having gained it and feared that I would never stop hating my body, much less ever hope to *like* it. All around me, I noticed women who I felt were thinner than me. I saw them sitting next to me in class, walking down the street, on billboards, in magazines, and in other areas of the media. I was frustrated by the knowledge of how my body used to look, disgusted with how my body presently looked, and horrified by the thought of what my body might become. I truly believed that I could not be happy or enjoy my life unless I lost weight. My preoccupation with food, dieting, and my body had completely taken over my life.

The Problem of Diet Culture

The most common (and most pervasive) driver of this sort of body idolatry is the diet industry, which constantly bombards us with the message that we need to change the way we eat and look. Therefore, if we have any hope of reconciling with our bodies, we first need to accept them; we need to surrender the compulsion to diet. But we can't stop dieting without also giving up the desire to alter our bodies. The whole point of most diets is to change how we look, which comes from a place of dissatisfaction. On the other hand, the truth of God's love sets us free to find our satisfaction in his love for us. If we continue to hold on to even the slightest hope that losing weight will meet our needs and longings, it will prevent us from experiencing the freedom and joy that result from knowing we are loved by God exactly as we are, exactly as he created us to be. We will continue to experience distracting thoughts about food, eating, and exercise until we can accept our bodies as God does. As Evelyn Tribole and Elyse Resch write, "As long as you are at war with your body, it will be difficult to be at peace with yourself and [with] food."[1]

Giving up a weight-loss ideal and working through fears surrounding our bodies are not easy by any means. Our culture makes it especially difficult to embrace body diversity because thin bodies are overwhelmingly valued above larger ones. In their book, Tribole and Resch explain how the world of fashion has distorted the cultural ideals of beauty. They discuss the influence of emaciated but renowned supermodels like Twiggy and Kate Moss and even point out that supposedly "plus-sized" fashion figures are often unhealthfully thin too: "When clothing giant, Guess, hired model Anna Nicole Smith," they write, "she made headlines in the fashion and news media because she was 'big.' Her weight was actually in the lower range of ideal according to 1990 U.S. height and weight charts!"[2] The more that thin models are celebrated and heavier women are criticized, the more likely it is that viewers of these advertisements will come to share the sentiment that smaller bodies are more beautiful than larger ones and develop feelings of shame and self-disgust for themselves unless they too are at a low weight.

From a young age, girls are trained to want to be thin: they receive admiration for appearing dainty and are often ostracized for developing womanly curves earlier than their peers. They hear their mothers talk about weight loss, see them consuming diet pills and powders, and watch them poke and prod at their own bodies. Our daughters see advertisements that use carefully positioned, thin models and read objectifying words and phrases scrawled across magazine pages. They are praised (or hear others being praised) for weight loss, for being small, or for looking thinner. These words are even used as compliments! When body fat is discussed in negative terms, it becomes something to fear for young children, and this is a view we internalize and carry with us into adulthood. Exposure to these advertisements and messages as adults reinforces the value of thinness in our minds.

Another way body fat and eating habits become objectified is through the language we use to describe rich food or leisurely activities. Desserts are described as "naughty" or "sinfully delicious," as though God condemns pleasure in eating or as if enjoying sweet treats is immoral. We refer to TV shows and afternoon naps as "guilty pleasures," but we never talk about the guilt, frustration, and anxiety behind the "after" picture in weight-loss comparisons. (Sure, we look thinner after a thirty-pound weight loss, but we feel awful.) As long as we use this language and continue to believe that something is wrong with our bodies as God created them, institutions are going to continue to keep trying to sell us thinness in quick, convenient, gimmicky packages, attempting to profit from our vulnerability.

Diets Sell Lies

Dieting is a key example of a practice that has the appearance of wisdom but doesn't truly have value. Diets are marketed as a means for weight loss, but the companies behind them are selling one of the most widely believed lies: that they can help us change our bodies for good. Not only are the vast majority of diet books written by non–health professionals, but almost none of them are actually based on quality scientific evidence. While many dieting regimes probably haven't been studied in depth, research has clearly demonstrated that *regardless of the nature of the diet plan*, dieting as a whole is an ineffective means of achieving long-term weight loss. In fact, most diets result in weight *gain*. Studies show that even if some dieters are able to maintain a weight loss for six to twelve months, most end up gaining it back—and then some—within four years.[3] Ultimately, dieting doesn't create weight loss; it does the opposite and promotes weight gain!

Many people also believe the lie that losing weight will make them feel happier and better about themselves, which is a driving force behind their decision to attempt a diet. Therefore, people come to associate dieting efforts with the pursuit of a better, more fulfilling life. I don't know about you, but most of the dieters I talk to are far from chipper—they are irritable, distracted, fatigued, and downright *hangry*. Being ten to twenty pounds above your "goal weight" is probably not affecting your life as much as the dieting industry has made you believe. Your body's shape and size don't make you any less funny, any less loving, or any less patient, kind, or beautiful. But dieting? That certainly does! Whenever we deprive ourselves of food, we are depriving ourselves of the energy that sustains us. We are depressing our moods, exhausting ourselves, and driving our minds to focus on everything we aren't eating instead of important things like relationships, school, work, and ministry.

Many times, our views of the reality of dieting are distorted by stories we read on the internet. Especially today, the web is overridden by blogs by "healthy living gurus" who share tips for wellness, weight loss, eating, and exercise. First of all, most of these bloggers are completely lacking in credentials. While I don't believe that you need to have a degree or any sort of formal training to rightfully share truth with others, it becomes much more likely that a person will advertise false, misleading, or dangerous information if they haven't received a thorough education in nutrition and medicine. A person might have achieved a particular weight-loss result through a certain protocol or set of steps, but that doesn't mean that it's safe, healthy, or advisable for others to do the same. Every person's body is unique, and that is why it's essential to consult a health professional before radically changing your eating and exercise patterns. Healthy living involves so much more than body weight, and neglecting sound medical advice to pursue weight loss can have devastating consequences.

Many of the radical dieting stories we hear don't share the difficult aspects of that person's journey, like the medical struggles they face as a result of weight loss or their actual health status. Rapid weight loss produces a loss of bone density and muscle, strains the kidneys and heart, and can cause potentially fatal electrolyte imbalances regardless of the person's original weight. These risks aren't only for people who start dieting when they are already thin—they are a risk for *everyone.* Even if the dieting effort is not prolonged, repeated cycles of weight loss and weight gain (such as those seen in yo-yo dieting) are actually more dangerous to a person's health than remaining the same weight. These fluctuations increase stress hormones, blood pressure, and the risk of heart attack, stroke, and diabetes. A well-known research endeavor called the Framingham Heart Study showed that weight cycling of this nature increases the overall death rate and elevates the risk of dying from heart disease to *twice the normal risk.*[4]

Another danger of recurrent dieting is the risk of developing fertility problems. Most of the women I talk with mention that they'd rather not have a period at all because monthly visits from Aunt Flo are inconvenient, uncomfortable, and sometimes embarrassing. I can't say I disagree, but I know that regular menstrual cycles are an important reflection of overall health. Usually when a woman isn't taking good care of herself, nonessential life functions like fertility are the first to be affected. Late or missing periods due to physical or emotional stress are pretty common, as are painful cramps, irritable moods, and other PMS symptoms. Even though most women experience these abnormalities on occasion, the "normalcy" of them doesn't mean that they're benign. Rather, menstrual irregularities are a huge problem. The World Health Organization estimates that up to 10 percent of women globally face fertility struggles—getting and staying pregnant.[5] This doesn't include the additional millions of women affected by other menstrual disorders.

I was somewhat of a late bloomer back in the day and didn't start my period until I was fourteen. Incidentally, this was close to the same time that I started restricting my diet. Because of my struggles with food and exercise and frequent weight changes, I can count on one hand the number of times I had my period as a teenager—I didn't start having regular cycles until I was in my twenties. It certainly was convenient at the time, but my missing period was a sign that my health was suffering even when I wasn't underweight. A woman doesn't need to be anorexic for unhealthy eating habits to affect her fertility.

Whenever a period is delayed or missing, there are changes in the balance of sex hormones in the body, most notably estrogen and proges-terone. When these hormones aren't in the proper range, the body starts to lose bone density. (This is why postmenopausal women often develop osteoporosis, which can lead to fractures, pain, and disfiguring postural changes.) The scariest part of this is that bone density loss is pretty much permanent—bone density peaks at around twenty-two years old, and any accelerated loss after that time sets a woman up for severe problems in the future. But bone loss isn't the only risk of low estrogen—it can also cause insomnia, migraines, depression, cardiovascular disease, fatigue, metabolic dysregulation, and weight gain, as well as infertility. While fertility problems can often be corrected under the care of a physician, sometimes the body permanently loses its ability to conceive and carry a baby. Physicians often prescribe birth control pills to stimulate monthly cycles, but these medications don't help promote pregnancy because they elicit *anovulatory* periods. (This means the woman has a period but isn't releasing an egg and therefore can't become pregnant.) Birth control pills prevent ovulation, so if a woman is not able to ovulate on her own, the birth control pill won't help her.

In college, my doctor prescribed birth control pills for me because of the risks associated with a missing period. However, I stopped taking them once I realized that although they were causing a monthly bleed, they weren't actually supporting my fertility. I wasn't looking to have a child at that time, but I knew having a family was something I wanted in the future. To start having my period normally, I needed to start eating more regular and balanced meals. Medications sometimes act as Band-Aids that cover up the underlying cause of a person's health problem, making it even more difficult to identify the real issue. As a result, we end up wasting time and money on "solutions" that aren't helping us at all.

Dieting Makes Sicker People

Dieters believe that subtracting weight and cutting back on what they eat will improve their health, but when we look at the facts, the numbers don't add up this way. The truth of the matter is that losing weight is ineffective at best and harmful at worst when it comes to promoting health. Everybody is at risk of health problems from dieting, not just individuals suffering from orthorexia or other eating disorders. Let's take a look at the research.

The current consensus among scientists shows that diets are ineffective in promoting long-term weight loss and paradoxically even lead to weight *gain* in most cases. Here's an example: A 2007 study published in the *American Journal of Psychology* reported that most dieters regain more weight than they lost during their time restricting their food intake. Likewise, even after the initial period of weight loss, the study showed no significant health improvement aside from weight change![6] Another study published in the *International Journal of Exercise Science* revealed that cycles of weight loss and regain (i.e., yo-yo dieting) disrupt normal physiology, slow the metabolism, increase fat percentage, and raise cholesterol levels, which dramatically increase the likelihood of a person developing cardiovascular disease. The researchers even noted that dieters faced an increased risk of developing type 2 diabetes and stroke.[7] This is all pretty alarming considering that most diets claim to improve these areas of wellness.

The media sensationalizes the supposed positive effects of dieting, and individual diet companies themselves continue to generate misleading headlines based on individual scientific findings that seldom play out as advertised. There's a big difference between research performed on mice in tightly controlled laboratory settings and the effects of restrictive dieting within the dynamic context of human life. Diet companies will continue to use these unsubstantiated conclusions as ammunition to support their cause, but it's a battle that the scientific community has already won. We just need to know where to look. Literature reviews consistently support conclusions like this one, given in a 2017 study of popular weight-loss strategies: "Despite the growing popularity of fad diets and exercise plans for weight loss, there are limited studies that actually suggest these particular regimens are beneficial and lead to long-term weight loss."[8] Once again, research has debunked the lie that dieting efforts offer significant health benefits.

Physical health isn't the only dimension at risk for dieters either. In their 2011 article published in the *Nutrition Journal*, researchers Linda Bacon and Lucy Aphramor point out that there is also a significant detriment to the mental and emotional wellness of dieters: "Concern has arisen that this weight focused paradigm is . . . damaging, contributing to food and body preoccupation, repeated cycles of weight loss and regain, distraction from other personal health goals and wider health determinants, reduced self-esteem, eating disorders, other health decrement, and weight stigmatization and discrimination."[9] The list continues, but ultimately their findings demonstrate that the best way to avoid these negative effects is to avoid focusing so much on the size and shape of our bodies. Adolescent health experts even recommend that parents not focus on weight or diet with their children but instead be mindful of the following considerations to encourage optimal mental and physical health:

1. "Discourage unhealthy dieting; instead, encourage and support the use of eating and physical activity behaviors that can be maintained on an ongoing basis";
2. "Promote a positive body image";
3. "Encourage more frequent, and more enjoyable, family meals";
4. "Encourage families to talk less about weight and do more at home to facilitate healthy eating and physical activity";
5. "Assume that overweight teens have experienced weight mistreatment and address this issue with teens and their families." (*Weight mistreatment* refers to bullying and/or discrimination on account of a person's body shape and size.)[10]

The healthiest thing we can do for ourselves and our families is reduce our focus on food, weight, and diet by building our attunement skills so that we can eat with the freedom that God desires for us. It's undeniably radical and countercultural, yet the above recommendations are supported by both health professionals and the Bible's expression of God's love for us. Focusing too much on dieting and food honors neither God nor ourselves, but exercising freedom in our eating honors both.

A Huge Waste

Diets not only fail to add anything of value to our lives; they also lead to wastefulness in very measurable ways. Whether a waste of time, a waste of money, or a waste of mental attention, they drain our resources in the meaningless pursuit of a smaller body. Christian circles have not been immune to the messaging of diet culture, with the rise of church-based weight-loss groups, "Christian" versions of diet books, and faith-forward fitness bloggers. They even go so far as to claim biblical support for their messaging, but the verses they cite are taken completely out of context. Although Paul shares an encouragement in writing, "I have fought the good fight, I have finished the race," the message of 2 Timothy 4:7 (ESV) has nothing to do with actual running. Contrary to (increasingly) popular belief, a toned physique is not a Christian virtue. God's love for us does not depend on the shapes of our bodies or the content of our dinners. While we certainly can and should seek to honor God in the way we approach food and health, if at any point our food-related concerns trump our knowledge of God's love, we're extremely mixed up. Even if we claim that we don't believe that the purpose of life is to chase beauty or weight loss, do our calendars, checkbooks, and mental lists tell a different story? Are we spending more on gym memberships, organic groceries, and meal-replacement shakes than on contributions to the church and missionaries? Ultimately, the call to realign our focus from food to God is meant not to denounce the value of health initiatives but rather to set us free from enslavement to the belief that we need those things in order to "earn" value in life. Pouring time, money, and energy into diet programs drains resources that could be better allocated toward things that actually do enrich our lives.

First of all, diet plans and products are extremely expensive. Most diets claim some sort of secret knowledge about an elusive ingredient, exercise, or method that will cause a fifty-pound weight loss in three days, cure every disease, make you instantly beautiful, free you from debt, and deliver you into spiritual nirvana. All you have to do is buy it—*problem solved*! Well, not so much. As we know, diets don't work like this. So investing in a dieting protocol is an outright waste of money. Even if the diet initially creates desirable results, it can't deliver in the long run, and these programs don't come with five-month money-back guarantees. Most diet plans aren't cheap, so they are big investments without a lot of return.

Despite failing to provide an effective solution, diet pills and powders are everywhere. Protein shakes, fiber bars, juice cleanses, and gluten-free products are also markedly more expensive than whole food items, which are of higher quality. Since foods in their natural form such as whole apples or chicken haven't been processed down into their individual components, they offer the same protein, vitamins, and other nutrients for significantly less money. Another way that money is lost on diets is with unused product. Many people give up on their diets before completion, and the remaining pills, powders, and packets end up unused because they are objectively less delicious than home-cooked meals. It's less common for someone to buy chicken and not cook it than it is for someone to buy protein powder and not use it. The "diet" versions of traditional products are also often more expensive but less satisfying. For example, for a dollar more at Jimmy John's, you can convert your sandwich into an "un-wich," which is their name for a sandwich without bread. In other words, you pay extra to receive less food.

Some diet plans capitalize on a sort of "whole food" approach, encouraging the consumption of certain types of foods that are often more expensive than their regular counterparts. For example, you can buy "Whole 30 compliant" bacon at Whole Foods and "keto-friendly" gummy bears at almost every health food store. In addition, Weight Watchers "points" are listed everywhere from online databases to foods themselves. While these diet programs don't necessarily require the purchase of a specific product or membership, the highly restrictive way of eating they require often warrants the purchase of pricier groceries. They also require an excessive amount of planning and preparation that effectively turns eating into a full-time job.

Following a diet—especially lifestyle diets like Whole 30, keto, and Weight Watchers—requires a significant investment of time and energy. With each new plan, a person needs to learn new food rules, plan out grocery lists, and practice complicated recipes, often with obscure and expensive ingredients, using up brain space and financial margin that might be better allocated elsewhere. In some ways, these programs really are more of a lifestyle than a diet—the time, energy, and effort required to comply with them completely take over a person's life, requiring extensive sacrifices that affect mental health, relationships, and more. And these diet-centered lifestyles are vastly different from a lifestyle characterized by joy, confidence, and freedom rooted in God's love.

This is all without even considering the time-consuming exercise requirements of many of these regimes. Of course, bodily movement is very important to wellness. But current research doesn't suggest that it's necessary to work out in a particular way—whether running a certain number of miles or lifting a certain amount of weight per week. Exercise takes on many different methods and forms and doesn't need to be strictly monitored or controlled. The same principles of intuition in eating can be applied to exercise: when the amount or use of movement in our lives is out of balance, whether too much or too little, our bodies respond. Lethargy, restlessness, poor sleep, and depressed mood are often symptoms of too little exercise, while anxiety, joint pain, fatigue, and extreme hunger may signal too much exercise. The best way to gauge a healthy and balanced amount of movement in your life is by learning how to listen to your body, not by subscribing to a beach body workout plan.

While we all benefit from regular exercise, an enormous variety of modalities are available to us. If lifting weights feels like torture, slaving away in the gym simply isn't necessary. There's no reason to exchange valuable hours of your life if you can receive the same benefit from other types of exercise that you truly enjoy, such as doing yoga or playing tennis. Being healthy doesn't mean we need to deprive ourselves of things we love. Likewise, there's no reason to force ourselves to eat foods we don't enjoy or engage in unpleasant or uncomfortable activities in order to be healthy.

Fighting the Wrong Fight

The health of our bodies deeply affects our daily lives. So naturally, when our health starts to suffer, our first inclination is usually to figure out what went wrong so we can fix it. But sometimes, these "health" problems have little to do with our bodies. We tend to zero in on nutrition and fitness as a means to manage something else that's going on—stressful work situations, broken families, heartache, or difficulty coping in general. When other areas of our lives feel out of control, sometimes we turn to dieting because all of its rules give us the illusion of stability and power. Sometimes we even end up blaming food for problems it didn't cause. Stomachache? Eliminate dairy. Acne? Avoid sugar. But then days or weeks later, the stomachaches or acne returns, so we blame another food group. As a result, our diets become more and more restrictive without eliciting any health benefits.

Anxiety, fear, and stress are especially difficult to separate from their very physical manifestations—stomachaches, acne, blood sugar fluctuations, or digestive problems. In our diet-obsessed culture, it's important to recognize how often our problems have nothing to do with food. Sometimes our bodies present symptoms of a seemingly unrelated problem that is much more difficult to identify. Of course, chronic digestive issues and depression are not entirely independent of physiology and food. But sometimes we blame food for these conditions when a closer look at physiology reveals that the root of the problem stretches much deeper than nutrition and lifestyle. Furthermore, sometimes when we manipulate our diets (by avoiding ingredients or starting a new diet), we compound our original symptoms, so rather than food causing our stomachaches, *stress* about food causes (or worsens) our stomachaches.

When it comes to health and body weight, many of us feel helpless or out of control. We fear that if we become too lax or let down our guard, our bodies will rebel against us by getting sick or gaining weight. But at the end of the day, our bodies are truly on our side. They don't hold secret vendettas against us, looking to make us miserable. Rather, we and our bodies share the common goal of trying to stay alive! Our bodies' natural tendency isn't to gain excessive weight or create uncontrollable appetites. In fact, when we fall into harmful habits, our bodies send us signals urging us to do something differently. The problem is that most of us have tuned out those signals—usually through dieting—and consequently don't understand how to work with our bodies instead of wrestling against them. When God created our bodies, he called them good. He designed them with love and gave them to us to cherish and respect. When we see our bodies as our enemies, we reject his gifts. But when we embrace our bodies and choose to be their allies, we can truly experience and *live out* God's love.

Missing Out on What Matters

Putting too great a focus on food and our bodies creates a sense of pre-occupation that distracts us from everything else God is doing in our lives. God designed food and exercise to empower us to enjoy life. Therefore, our approach to nutrition and fitness should support our lifestyles—not completely take them over. Whenever we allow something to overwhelm our lives, whether through our thoughts or actions, we end up missing out on what really matters. Pursuing food and exercise is not our ultimate purpose in life, and when our lives become skewed toward those things, we ultimately suffer. This is true even if we are pursuing those things to avoid suffering (such as from poor health). In her reflection on Whole 30, a popular, monthlong elimination diet, D. L. Mayfield writes, "We are a nation of overeaters and dieters, of workout obsessives and 'fat acceptance' advocates, and I find myself somewhat lost in the perspectives on what it means to feel good and look good. I want to be healthy and happy, but I want it to be based in something deeper than appearances."[11] Mayfield is not alone. So often, we turn to food (or control of food) as a means for satisfaction, purpose, or meaning. But our true purpose in life is found in something much deeper than our diets.

When I finally recovered from nearly a decade of disordered eating and obsessive exercise, I felt lost for a while. Without dieting, I didn't know who I was, and that terrified me. But as the fog of calories that had clouded my mind for so long slowly started to fade, I found myself noticing, pondering, and becoming fascinated by things I had otherwise completely ignored. One morning, as I gazed out the window during breakfast, I realized right then and there that I was seeing colors for the first time. I had spent so many of my days in a state of avoidance, thinking about food and fitness so I could ignore the reality of my life. Even though I'd shown up every day, I'd missed majestic sunrises that covered the world in shining gold; the stark contrast of my black-and-white dog against the cheerfully green grass; the way that creeks, ponds, and puddles reflected the mesmerizing blue sky. Life was beautiful, and I had missed so much of it. Life without dieting—the beautiful life God created—was breathtaking.

I even started noticing how good it felt to be in a body that wasn't being starved, overstuffed, or punished with exercise. In recovery, I learned about the satisfying relief that comes from eating before the point of ravenousness, the pleasant comfort of fullness after enjoying a tasty and nourishing meal, and the freedom in taking a deep breath without simultaneously trying to suck in my belly. I learned how invigorating a slow, simple stretch can be and that when I rested appropriately, my knees didn't hurt. Beyond the comfort of a full belly, giving up dieting allowed me to experience the joy of a fulfilled heart, satisfied by a deep and intimate relationship with the God who loved me so much that he chose to give me life.

Have your diet restrictions caused you to miss out on joy, peace, or purpose? Has dieting led you to refrain from dining out with friends or attending food-related celebrations? Have you ever skipped out on enjoying a piece of your birthday cake for the sake of weight loss? Or turned down social invitations because you had a strict exercise schedule to follow? Have you ever weighed yourself and found that the number on the scale ruined your mood for the entire day? Or spurred you into a

Every day!

cloud of shame and guilt? Unfortunately, these experiences are extremely common in our society, especially among women. The pressure to be thin and our fears about disease and death drive us to take extreme approaches that detract from our lives. Our intentions all along were to make our lives *better*, right? Major oops!

As humans, fearfully and wonderfully made and deeply loved by God, our value cannot be measured by numbers. We are so much more than calories, pounds, miles, or reps. Our freedom in Christ invites us into a life of abundance, not a life of shame, enslavement to food rules, or fear about health and longevity. God put each of us on this earth with a purpose far greater than fitting into a certain pants size. Our health problems in modern America don't totally result from what we do or don't eat; rather, they are the result of a break in the connection between the mind, body, and spirit that God created for us in the beginning. However, that connection truly can be healed. We each were born with the tools for doing so, and they still reside inside of us; we just need to learn how to use them again.

CHAPTER FOUR

Health at Every Size

You Don't Have to Be Thin to Be Healthy

While self-image plays at least a partial role in motivating most diets, some of us have body weight concerns that stem from the desire to honor God by taking care of our health (i.e., to "exercise good stewardship over our bodies"). While each hold some degree of responsibility for our individual well-being, most people have a flawed idea of what health actually means due to the media's sensationalist portrayal of the relationship between weight and wellness. Despite what magazine headlines might lead us to believe, we can't photoshop bodies into becoming healthier. So far, we've unpacked a number of problems caused by a dieting mindset, but the ones that require the most attention are those that affect our health. The relationship between health and body size (or lack thereof) is too significant to ignore. So it's time to clear up some commonly held false beliefs about the role of body fat in human health. Instead of focusing our attention on meaningless measurements like body mass index (BMI), we'll explore a science-based, alternative view of physical wellness that avoids both condemnation and complete abandonment in eating.

A Bigger Body Doesn't Mean You're Unhealthy

In college, I spent a few months living with a family friend who followed an objectively *very* healthy diet with impressive consistency. Her eating habits were like those you might expect from a doctor or nutrition professional: She ate lean, fresh protein sources, vegetables at every meal, few refined grain products, and maybe a cup or two of coffee each day. She rarely ate sweets and never kept snacks like chips or crackers around. She also rode her bike to and from work each day and went for long runs on weekends. During the time I lived with her, she ran two 5K races and a half marathon. The year prior, she'd participated in marathons and long-distance bicycle races both locally and abroad. In addition to distance running, she was actively involved in CrossFit and enjoyed competitive power lifting as a hobby. (Impressive, right?) I knew from talking to her and living with her that her eating and exercise habits weren't fads or halfhearted efforts she ditched after a few months. She lived her life like an athlete, through and through.

The interesting thing about this friend, however, is that others might look at her and assume that she ate and exercised very differently than she did. Her entire life, she'd lived in a larger body—one that was classified as overweight according to traditional measures, like BMI. But she never let outward appearances or stereotypes get in the way of nourishing her body and pursuing athletic goals. So was she healthy? I firmly believe the answer is a huge, resounding *yes*. The research overwhelmingly shows that the factors that influence health aren't numbers like weight or calories but consistent behaviors over time, and she had a lengthy track record of health-promoting behaviors.

The unhealthiest I'd ever seen my friend was when she was pregnant with her first child and suffered hyperemesis gravidarum, an extreme version of morning sickness, which caused her to lose more than thirty pounds in one month due to nausea and vomiting. Some people—sadly, even physicians—might have seen that weight loss on paper (pregnancy aside) and celebrated it in the name of health. But there is absolutely nothing healthy about skipping meals, throwing up, and dropping weight so quickly—no matter a person's initial size. Another friend of mine quickly lost weight in the same way after becoming infected with a gastrointestinal disease she contracted while on a mission trip. She was bedridden for months and even ended up needing surgery because of it. I witnessed her receiving numerous compliments for her weight loss, and each time my heart sank because I knew that there was absolutely nothing healthy about what she'd gone through. Body fat is not a bad thing, and there's nothing inherently praiseworthy about having less of it.

An individual's external appearance doesn't accurately represent what's going on *inside*, and I'm not just referring to character qualities. Regardless of their weight, a person can have excellent results on blood tests and physical diagnostic exams that measure internal health. A person in a larger body may have healthy blood pressure, cholesterol, and other laboratory measures despite an elevated BMI. At the same time, a thin person may have poor results on these same tests or may suffer from other health problems as a result of their eating, exercise, or other lifestyle behaviors. During my time in recovery for my eating disorder, I met friends who had been hospitalized for complications from both starving and binge eating, some of which nearly killed them.

In clinical practice, measuring a person's weight alone doesn't provide a direct measure of their health risks. Of course, if a person has a relatively higher weight and also eats only donuts, the likelihood is high that the person would be unwell and have a higher risk of developing disease. But the issue in such cases is behavior, not body mass. In my own practice, I've treated skinny patients for high cholesterol and clinically obese patients for low blood pressure (a condition usually associated with smaller-bodied individuals). Contrary to what the media portrays, a thinner body does not prevent chronic diseases, and a larger body doesn't cause them.

This is especially true in the case of lifestyle stress, a phenomenon that afflicts an extremely large proportion of the American population. Countless studies demonstrate that long-term exposure to stress leads to weight gain, and not just because of emotional eating. An article published in the *International Journal of Obesity* describes a study of parents whose children had been diagnosed with cancer. Compared to parents of healthy children, these understandably stressed parents consumed fewer calories but gained more weight over three months.[1] Other studies of individuals in high-stress situations have yielded similar results, including findings of increased abdominal fat levels in addition to generalized weight gain.[2] For many individuals, rather than weight gain causing their physical symptoms, the rising number on the scale is simply another symptom of a different underlying problem, such as chronic stress or an undiagnosed disease. In fact, focusing so much on weight can distract doctors from uncovering the root cause of their patients' symptoms.

One of my friends recently received a weight-loss recommendation from her doctor when he saw her elevated cholesterol level. She'd gained about twenty pounds in the last five years due to a combination of menopause and a foot injury that interfered with her exercise routine. "I don't understand why that's his best advice," she said, frustrated, "when my weight is the only thing that's changed since my last visit! My cholesterol was high even when I was thin! He never mentioned weight loss then, but now that I've filled out a little, it feels like all he sees is the number on the scale." Her doctor even refused to run further diagnostic tests until she lost the weight she had gained. Sadly, her story isn't unique. Working in health care, I hear accounts like this all the time. I've also noticed that many of my patients acknowledge their size in some capacity when they come into the office for completely unrelated ailments. One patient with a swollen ankle said, "I know I need to lose weight, but this can't be just because I'm heavy." She was absolutely right—her torn ligament and avulsion fracture were in no way a consequence of her body size. Her injury had nothing to do with her weight and everything to do with the fact that she'd slipped on a patch of ice. I've also heard stories of physicians who dismissed their patients' concerns of swelling or pain on account of their weight, letting blood clots, thyroid disease, and other pathologies continue undiagnosed for weeks, months, or even years.

Standards of care concerning body weight are slow to change. Currently, the norm in physicians' offices is to weigh patients at every visit and counsel them about weight loss if their BMI is out of the recommended range. Even though the Centers for Disease Control and Prevention (CDC) acknowledges that BMI should not be used as a diagnostic tool,[3] physicians still plaster infographics across the walls of their clinics. The charting software used during my internship even flagged patients whose BMI fell into the "at risk of becoming overweight" category—even those who were gaining weight because they were pregnant.

Why measure something that isn't clinically relevant? Why discuss weight loss with a patient when body weight isn't their problem? It's likely these measurements are taken not because they are helpful or informative but simply out of routine. An article published in the *British Medical Journal* describes the issue perfectly. Authors Susan Wooley and David Garner write, "It could be said that the main evidence for the value of dieting is that health professionals continue to prescribe it. Inertia feeds on itself, failure to change coming to serve as a silent argument that no change is needed. . . . Dieting not only fails the criterion of being without risk but has been implicated in increased morbidity and mortality in several large studies. Dieting often has negative effects on psychosocial functioning and can lead to eating disorders such as binge eating disorder and even bulimia nervosa. Finally, dietary treatments are costly, unpleasant, and, when they fail, tend to damage self-esteem."[4] In other words, dieting harms patients, increasing their risk of developing eating disorders and even elevating the risk of death! Yet doctors still prescribe weight-loss diets because that's what they know. They were taught to do it in school, they see their colleagues doing it, and it's built into their routine. Recommending weight loss to an overweight patient is the only solution they know of, regardless of whether other options exist. When the only tool you have is a hammer, everything starts to look like a nail.

Healthy Weight Set Points

I'm not trying to negate the fact that excess weight can carry health risks. This is a widely understood truth in modern medicine, but it has also been blown out of proportion. The key word in describing the relationship between weight and health is *excessive*. *Excessively* high weight carries risk—not five to ten pounds. Many people have adopted an inaccurate view of healthy body weight. They also fail to recognize that different people have different weight set points. This term refers to the natural shape and size of each of our bodies, which is genetically determined and unique to each of us. Your individual physique is never going to be the same as that of Kate Middleton, Kim Kardashian, or your best friend. You also are never going to have the same physiologic propensity to look like you did ten years ago, and you will likewise settle into a somewhat different shape and size ten years from now.

Trying to establish a physique that isn't your own body's weight set point is not only physically harmful but also extremely difficult. If a woman needs to follow an extremely restrictive diet, cut calories, and exercise excessively in order to maintain her weight—even a healthy weight on the low end of the spectrum—that weight is likely not where her body wants to be. On the other hand, respecting and accepting the genetically determined shape and size of her body will help her easily maintain both her weight *and* her sense of well-being. A woman who has found her body's weight set point doesn't restrict her diet, moves her body regularly, and doesn't worry about the nitty-gritty details of her appearance. She also enjoys a variety of satisfying foods in sufficient quantities to maintain high energy levels while completing her daily tasks. Your weight set point is going to be different from your neighbor's weight set point, but it might be similar to—within twenty pounds of—that of your mother (or your sister if you have one).

Your weight set point is determined by your DNA, just like shoe size, bust size, or hair color, and it's the size and shape your body naturally wants to be. Sure, you can shove your feet into shoes that are too small, or dye your hair, or starve yourself to be a few pants sizes smaller, but at the end of the day, your genes are still your genes. Just as some of us carry more muscle or have a larger bust size, some of us weigh more or less or have a higher or lower body fat percentage. It's the way we were made. In addition, our weight set points might change every couple of decades due to normal hormonal variations throughout our lives. A ten-year-old girl generally has a different weight set point than she will as a sixteen-year-old. Women who have never given birth will naturally have a different shape and size than they would if they were postpartum. Weight fluctuations are normal. Just as it's unfair to expect our bodies to look like those of other women, it's unrealistic to expect our bodies to stay exactly the same throughout our lives.

When your weight is outside your own individual weight set point, your body will undergo metabolic changes to help you return to a healthy range. Your appetite will automatically increase or decrease, and you will burn through energy either more or less efficiently depending on which direction your body wants to go. Symptoms of being at a weight below your body's healthy range include sleepiness, feeling cold all the time, irritability, low sex drive, irregular or absent menstrual cycles, struggling to prevent weight gain, depression, thin hair, and dry skin to name a few. On the other hand, symptoms of being above your body's natural weight can include fatigue, feeling overheated, a red face, breathlessness, insomnia, and anxiety. These are not diagnostic criteria, meaning that you can't determine whether you're at your weight set point based on these criteria. The only way to fall into your own personal healthy weight range is to eat intuitively for a long enough time to arrive at that healthy place.

However, I can tell you definitively that if you're actively restricting your food intake, binge eating regularly, exercising excessively (more than an hour per day), not exercising at all, or sleeping fewer than seven hours each night, you are not taking care of your body well and likely are not at a stable or sustainable weight. Undereating and undersleeping can leave you either above or below your body's weight set point—and if you're starving your body of food or rest, you're definitely not healthy. Once you start taking care of yourself, however, your body weight will eventually stabilize. You'll know you're at this point when, after a pattern of honoring your hunger and fullness cues, eating a variety of foods, and resting enough, your weight stops changing and your clothes still fit despite the complete absence of any attempt to externally control your weight. In some ways, you won't know you're on the right path until you've arrived at your destination.

The Myth of Unhealthy Food

Author Michael Pollan famously writes in his book *In Defense of Food* that the key to balanced eating is simple: "Eat food. Not too much. Mostly plants."[5] He elaborates on this, saying that origin differentiates "real" food from the alternative. Plants grown in the ground are real food, he argues, whereas products *made in a plant* (i.e., a factory) are not real food and should not be eaten. This perspective perfectly represents the notion of "clean" versus "unclean" or "healthy" versus "unhealthy" food. But I'm here to tell you that the only unclean food is the *unwashed* kind—with literal chunks of dirt on it. The official position held by the Academy of Nutrition and Dietetics (ANAD) is that all foods can fit into a healthy diet. In their formal statement on nutrition, ANAD authors urge against an all/none, good/bad, right/wrong view toward nutrition, noting the unhelpfulness of such a perspective: "When too much emphasis is given to a single food or food component, confusion and controversy can hinder, rather than facilitate, consumers in adopting healthy dietary patterns."[6] They explain how early nutrition studies identified a causative relationship between saturated fat and heart disease that has since been disproven and how substituting these with foods low in saturated fat, such as egg whites or soy-based products, can result in nutrient deficiencies. That same risk isn't present with regular, full-fat cheeseburgers. We don't need replacements because there is nothing wrong with the original design.

Speaking of cheeseburgers, foods like these generally have a bad reputation in the diet community. Aside from their high levels of saturated fat (which has been proven to be less problematic than initially thought), burgers, fries, and similar items are criticized for being high in calories. But contrary to popular belief, calories are not a bad thing. Calories are units of energy, and energy keeps us alive. Foods high in energy are also often high in the vital nutrients we need to thrive. Low-calorie foods are not necessarily healthier. Most diet food products are not only void of energy but void of other nutrients too. If we eat air-puffed cereal that is very low in calories but also low in vitamins, minerals, and staying power, is it even worth eating?

Another highly controversial number on nutrition labels is grams of sugar. The media loves to talk about the harmful, addicting, and inflammatory effects of sugar. But again, these sensationalized claims completely lack scientific validity. Let's talk about research for a moment. Thousands of new studies are published every day in the field of health, and most simply acknowledge one-dimensional findings. For example, a team of researchers observed in their laboratories that when rats eat sugar, their brains release dopamine.[7] The researchers then published their findings and shared them with the greater scientific community. Early results such as these are strictly observational and carry no weight on their own. The next necessary step is for more research to be done to assess the significance of the results.

However, a number of journalists read a summary of the study and concluded that since drugs also create a dopamine response in the brain, sugar must be addictive, just like drugs. Everyone started talking about this "revolutionary finding," and before long, sugar became the next demonized food additive. But other scientists read the studies too. More studies were conducted, reviewed, and compared against each other, and the ultimate consensus was completely unremarkable. A review article published in the *European Journal of Nutrition* concludes, "We find little evidence to support sugar addiction in humans, and findings from the animal literature suggest that addiction-like behaviors, such as bingeing, occur only in the context of intermittent access to sugar. These behaviors likely arise from intermittent access to sweet tasting or highly palatable foods, not the neurochemical effects of sugar."[8] Stated simply, the rats only overate sugar when they were deprived of it. When they were offered regular access to food, they ate normally.

There are many limitations to the sweeping claims made about "dangerous," "toxic," or "addictive" ingredients, but the emotional nature of these claims distracts readers from recognizing those limitations. Instead of pointing the public toward accurate study findings, journalists use these sensationalized headlines to perpetuate false ideas about harmful food—all for the sake of clickbait. Sure, sugar seems addictive, but only in extreme cases. Yes, saturated fat poses health risks, but only when it is consumed in absurdly high quantities. Even water can be deadly when we drink too much of it. Ultimately, the notion of "unhealthy food" is a myth. The detailed composition of a person's individual meals is far less important to their well-being than their eating patterns over time. Eating a brownie won't ruin your health, regardless of how much you weigh.

Lifestyle Is Everything

As a health care provider, I see it as my duty to uncover the overall patterns in my patients' lives rather than focusing on minute details like whether they ate dessert yesterday. Not only are behavior patterns valuable in understanding the complexities of a patient's condition, but overall changes in lifestyle habits are often the most effective treatment options in managing chronic health problems. This is especially true for more common conditions like cardiovascular disease and diabetes. Sometimes these lifestyle changes result in weight loss, but they don't always; other times they result in weight gain. While a patient's weight is not completely inseparable from his or her behaviors, the scale isn't the most important place to look.

A 2015 study released by the Department of Health and Human Services regarding heart disease outcomes demonstrates that for both heavyset and thin individuals, fitness level is far more important than body weight.[9] Exercise results in health benefits not because of its effects on body mass but because it helps control stress, improves sleep, lowers the risk of heart disease, supports blood sugar control, and elevates mood—among countless other positive effects. Other important lifestyle behaviors that dramatically impact a person's well-being regardless of weight include smoking, use of alcohol and caffeine, psychological stress, and even safety habits such as seat belt or bike helmet use. Especially with regard to the latter factors, the effects of dieting and weight loss cannot outweigh those of risky behaviors.

At the End of the Day, Remember Who Is in Control

When I was a newly licensed driver, my understandably concerned father would always warn me to drive "defensively." By this he meant I should look out for people who might be distracted or any deer that might choose to cross the road at inopportune times. If someone else had blown through a stop sign or crossed the median and involved me in an accident, it would not have been my fault. Sometimes accidents just happen.

But with winter driving (with which I have much experience, having lived in the Midwest my entire life), the lines between "my fault" and "not my fault" aren't as clear. Let's suppose I were to hit a patch of ice, lose control of my car, slide off the road, and collide with a tree. Would the accident have been my fault? It's hard to say for sure—maybe I should have been driving more slowly. But even if I had been driving more slowly, I still might have lost control of my car. Of course, there is wisdom to be applied to this sort of driving situation—both traveling too slowly and traveling too quickly can be dangerous, and accidents happen even when driving at an optimal speed.

Some principles of defensive driving can be applied to preventative health care. We are very fortunate in today's day and age to have a well-rounded understanding of the interplay between nutritional adequacy and disease risk. Completely ignoring nutrition recommendations can put us at a very significant risk for developing potentially fatal illnesses like diabetes and heart disease. But at the same time, dedicating too much thought, time, and energy to preventing disease can breed fear, anxiety, and stress, which not only spiritually damage us but wreak measurable havoc on our physical health. Likewise, we can cause nutritional imbalances by engaging in extreme eating patterns even if we were doing so to *prevent* health problems. There is a point at which the pursuit of healthy eating becomes unhealthy, just like driving too cautiously can actually put us at risk. That's where faith comes into play: we cannot control every aspect of our lives. But God can, and he promises to work all things for our good (Romans 8:28). Although we might feel frustrated at times by our lack of control over our bodies, this can also be extremely freeing. Intuitive eating allows us to put the responsibility back into God's hands so that we can set worry aside and rest instead in the comfort of his truth and love.

We Don't Need Diets to Be Healthy

Contrary to what many dieters claim, we can improve our health without losing any weight at all and also without creating a psychoemotional disturbance in our relationship with food.[10] Rather than changing our diets, we can reduce our risk of chronic illness and improve our mood by changing our *approach* to food. But first and foremost, to heal our relationship with food, we must refuse to diet in the first place. From a clinical perspective, the proof is in the pudding: randomized controlled trials indicate that a medical approach rooted in the health at every size (HAES) philosophy is associated with statistically and clinically relevant improvements in physiological measures (e.g., blood pressure, blood lipids), health behaviors (e.g., eating and activity habits, dietary quality), and psychosocial outcomes (such as self-esteem and body image) and that HAES achieves these health outcomes more successfully than weight-loss treatments and without the contraindications associated with a weight focus.[11] Ultimately, we don't need to become vegan, start eating low-carb, or begin a Whole 30 regime to reduce our risk of disease, lose weight, or help us "feel better" in our bodies.

Humans made up the definition of "overweight," not God. Body weight (and even health) is not a black-and-white issue. We tend to consider being "overweight" a bad thing because we are told that such a state will set us up for physical health problems. We have even come to associate *morality* with health, but this is not God's viewpoint. Believing that we are bad, wrong, or in any way less-than because of the size, shape, or health status of our bodies is believing a lie. God created each of us with unfathomable love and kindness, intentionally knitting together each of our unique bodies. The beauty of diversity is that we have tall and short, blonde and brunette, and blue-eyed and green-eyed and brown-eyed brothers and sisters of all shapes, sizes, and colors. The human body is a beautiful and magnificent creation and is a gift from God to each of us. There is glory in every single body of every shape and size, and we can cultivate health in such diversity too—no weight loss necessary.

CHAPTER FIVE

Eating with Freedom

God's Design for the Role of Food in Human Life

God desires for us to approach food with freedom. But for many of us, it has been years, maybe decades, since we last experienced food freedom—if we've ever experienced it at all. Many of my patients say they can't even remember a time when they didn't view food in moralistic terms or without constant diet chatter whirring in the back of their minds. For most of the women I speak with, the idea of food freedom is so foreign, it's inconceivable. It's not uncommon for a patient to say to me, "I'm sorry, but I can't even picture what a diet-free approach to food would look like."

In practice, I find that the best way to describe intuitive eating to my patients is by first explaining what it *isn't*. Of course, food and body image struggles look different in each of our lives, but the majority of individuals fall into one of three general categories of nonintuitive eaters: yo-yo dieters, fitness gurus, or mind*less* eaters. As you read through the descriptions below, think of how your own habits compare. Then, as we start uncovering what it means to be an intuitive eater, consider the differences between this and your own life, paying special attention to the areas that exhibit the most disparity.

What Kind of Eater Are You?

1. The Yo-Yo Dieter

Anna had always been considered overweight. She started attending Weight Watchers with her mom in elementary school and learned how to carefully monitor her eating by counting points. As she reached high school, she started trying other types of diets as well, ranging from low carb to vegan to full-blown fasting. She usually would be successful in losing a few pounds with these attempts, but after a few weeks, she would find herself secretly binge eating all the foods she'd been so meticulously avoiding. By the time she graduated from college, Anna had completely given up on her body. She felt uncomfortable in her skin, guilty for eating almost anything, and tired of her yo-yo cycle: salads for lunch and sleeves of cookies at midnight.

2. The Fitness Guru

Sam was proud to call herself a clean eater. She had been an active and athletic individual throughout her childhood and twenties and even earned a degree in kinesiology from a well-known university. She considered herself a self-educated nutrition expert as well—always attuned to the latest scientific studies about food and fitness. Sam was usually very careful to avoid "unhealthy foods." She was happy to celebrate birthdays at work but never sampled the cake, donuts, or bags of chips her coworkers would bring in to share. She also rarely ate at restaurants because her strict diet plan couldn't accommodate the high-calorie meals or the unknown ingredients. As a result, Sam regularly found herself turning down invitations to social events and usually would hit the gym instead.

3. The Mindless Eater

Jordan was a fit and active adult in his younger years, but once he and his wife had children, he started gaining weight. His job was stressful, and he'd usually numb out his frustration with deadlines and coworkers by snacking. He would find himself taking numerous trips to the vending machine throughout the day, ordering delivery for lunch, and then finishing an entire bag of chips before bed. Jordan was always munching, always finishing the food in front of him, and sometimes finishing his wife's food as well—he couldn't fathom the idea of letting leftovers go to waste. Instead, he found them accumulating at his waist.

Do any of these anecdotes resonate with you? Like Anna, do you constantly find yourself yo-yo dieting, stuck in a restriction-and-binge cycle? Or are you like Sam, committed to health and wellness to the point that it is all-consuming? Or finally, are you like Jordan, always eating without much regard to hunger and fullness and seeking convenience and comfort over quality? Most of you reading this book will reflect one of these eating patterns: frustrated and confused, obsessively meticulous, or seeking comfort to the point of numbness. There is also a fourth option, however: the free, intuitive eater.

Intuitive eaters, unlike Anna or Sam, don't pay attention to dieting specifics. They don't count calories, carbohydrates, or Weight Watchers points, and they don't see food as good or bad. Instead, they are closely attuned to what their bodies are telling them. Unlike Jordan, they don't eat when they aren't hungry, don't finish the food on their plates out of compulsion, and are more conscientious of food quality rather than convenience. For people who have been dieting for decades, the idea of exercising freedom in eating can seem very strange. Our whole lives, we have been told that we need to rely on meal plans, food pyramids, or tracking apps to tell us how, when, and how much to eat. We've been given neat, clean boxes to fill with serving sizes, recommended daily allowances, and daily values that we are encouraged to honor. The concept of intuitive eating, however, offers a framework that is much more flexible.

Intuitive Eating

The term *intuitive eating* refers to the process of feeding ourselves according to our body signals. With intuitive eating, all foods—and I really do mean all foods—fit, and a person uses internal cues to guide their food choices. Eating intuitively means making satisfying choices informed by knowledge of hunger, fullness, and how different foods make us feel, all without creating external rules. It also means using food as it was designed to be used (i.e., as fuel) and *not* using it to numb away feelings, satisfy our social needs, manipulate the size and shape of our bodies, or substitute the role of God in our lives. When we eat intuitively, we can fully embrace God's freedom, love, and grace when it comes to our bodies and how we view them. In practice, intuitive eating is the antithesis of dieting. While diets create numerous rules about food, intuitive eating has only one: there are no rules. Intuitive eating allows us to make choices about what, when, and how much to eat based on what our bodies tell us, whereas dieting determines what, when, and how much we eat by a schedule or a set of numbers (e.g., calories, Weight Watchers points, carbohydrate grams). Diets also ignore factors like hunger, satisfaction, and enjoyment of food, whereas intuitive eating embraces them.

In the beginning stages of intuitive eating, many of my patients fear that once they start letting themselves eat according to their cravings, they'll never stop. If you're worried about that too, I totally get it. This is exactly the type of fear mongering the diet industry uses—making us believe that we can't trust our bodies and therefore need to diet. But in these moments, as I advise my patients, remind yourself that God designed your body intelligently and intentionally. You can trust your body because you can trust the God who made it. He knew what he was doing, and he gave you hunger signals, fullness cues, cravings, and taste preferences for a reason. Your sweet tooth wasn't a mistake.

Sure, some people crave sweets more than others. My husband, for example, could enjoy life just fine if he never ate dessert again. But keep in mind that intuitive eating looks a little different for everyone. Each person has different energy and exercise needs, and we can't meet these needs with a one-size-fits-all approach. From work schedules, to home life, to person-to-person taste preferences, food fits into different lives in different ways. However, all intuitive approaches to eating consistently follow a few themes. These themes have rung true in my own recovery and are concepts I strive toward today as an intuitive eater. Together, we'll walk through these themes and guidelines before diving into more specifics—and practical tips—for embracing your food freedom. Let's get started:

1 **Surrendering the hope that a diet will make our lives better.**
   First things first: to eat intuitively, we have to give up dieting.
   Giving up dieting means choosing goals for ourselves that
   aren't centered on weight loss and consequently not using food
   as a means for changing our bodies. It means recognizing that
   our value and worth don't come from our bodies, and that
   food freedom and expressing kindness toward our bodies can
   improve our lives in ways that dieting never could. Practically,
   it also means resisting the urge to cut out entire food groups,
   read diet magazines, or participate in extreme behavior with
   food. (By extreme behavior, I'm referring to black-and-white,
   all-or-nothing behavior, such as restricting eating to certain
   times, skipping meals, or creating limitations based on calories,
   grams of nutrients, or other numbers.) In doing so, we actively
   remind ourselves that diets have failed to help us in the past
   and will not help us in the future either.

2 **Eating when we're hungry for food and not eating when we're
   hungry for something else.** Intuitive eating means allowing
   ourselves to eat if we're hungry at night, even if we already feel
   like we've eaten too much that day. It means choosing to eat
   breakfast even though we know we'll be eating a rich meal at
   lunch, but it also means not stuffing away our feelings after a
   hard day at work with a whole bag of potato chips (or chocolate

chips). By identifying what our bodies, minds, and souls truly need and responding in kind, we can care for ourselves most effectively. Developing this kind of self-awareness takes work, and in the next chapter, we will discuss the process of learning to identify needs so that we can cultivate a practice of self-care that honors our hearts, our minds, and our bodies, giving us plenty of next steps to take along the way.

3 **Getting rid of "good" and "bad" labels for food.** Intuitive eating means seeing cookies and kale as of equal importance in life even though they're not of equal nutritional value. It means enjoying an ice cream cone because it's delicious and fun and also eating salad because it keeps our bodies feeling amazing. The phrase in intuitive eating that describes this practice is "giving ourselves unconditional permission to eat." We've touched on some of these concepts already, but we will be discussing this process in practice even more in chapter 8.

4 **Enjoying all the delicious things about food and then putting down our forks when we're satisfied.** I hate cauliflower, so I don't eat it; but broccoli, when cooked right, is one of my all-time favorite foods. (Yes, seriously!) So when I'm eating broccoli, or buttered toast, or breaded chicken, I'm fully there—eyes, ears, mouth, nose, and all. I turn off the TV, put down my phone, and bring my whole self to the table. Cultivating this sense of awareness allows me to recognize when I'm satisfied and then stop eating. Unlike my dieting days, in which eating pizza almost always led to binge eating pizza, now as an intuitive, free eater, I am satisfied with just one or two slices. I'll be talking more about satisfaction and awareness of body signals in chapter 7.

5 **Ignoring the people who say otherwise.** For me, honoring my freedom to eat means unfollowing Instagram influencers who post diet talk on their pages and asking friends not to discuss their food rules. It means telling my brain to knock it

off when I find myself fantasizing about becoming Paleo or vegan or something else that's unsustainable and unnecessary without a medical reason, and choosing not to watch health documentaries on Netflix. In practice, I refer to this process as guarding our hearts, and I will explain it more fully in chapter 10.

6 **Eating a variety of foods.** I feel crummy when I only eat kale, but I also feel crummy when I only eat cookies. So I try to fill my plate with colorful, fresh food and choose flavors I enjoy. I pair carbs with protein to keep my blood sugar from dropping at 2 p.m., and I include veggies in most of my meals because they make me feel good and I know my body needs them. At the same time, I always say yes to cookies if they will make my taste buds happy. But when I'm not really craving cookies, I joyfully turn them down. Eating a variety of delicious and nutritious foods is an important piece of the wellness puzzle.

With intuitive, freedom-based eating, we sense our hunger and then permit ourselves to eat any food in any amount necessary to feel satisfied. Free eaters don't rely on external measures such as grams of carbohydrates in making food choices but instead rely on factors such as taste, pleasure, satisfaction, and knowledge about how the food makes them feel. Nutrition comes into consideration, but not to the point that it is prohibitive—there are no "shoulds" or "should nots" in intuitive eating. Rather, an intuitive eater has full power and autonomy over his or her ability to make food choices.

Think about how you currently make decisions about food. What influences your choices? Do you consider what you've already eaten that day? Do you pay attention to information you've heard on television, seen on billboards, or read on social media? Do you think about your body's shape and size, shame yourself, or try to use food to manipulate your appearance? These are common habits, likely because that's what we've been taught all our lives. But they don't help us take better care of ourselves. These food rules and the subsequent level of nutritional misunderstanding make eating a stressful experience. When God created humans, he never intended for eating to be such a difficult task. It was supposed to sustain our lives, not drain them! Food is a gift, and it is meant to be enjoyed.

Diets Lead to Condemnation, but God's Love Leads to Freedom

Many of my patients express concern about whether it's appropriate to eat foods the media deems unhealthy. They worry that they are taking liberties with their health by consuming French fries, donuts, or candy bars and consequently dishonoring God. They've been told all their lives that these foods are harmful—even *sinful* in their deliciousness—and feel that they should strive to follow a "cleaner diet," but God's design is for us to enjoy abundant and diverse diets for the sake of our own well-being.

One of the best examples of an intentional diet imbalance that is contrary to God's original design is the ketogenic diet. This diet is extremely low in carbohydrates, which forces the body to use a specific type of sugar, called ketones, for fuel. Ketones are produced during the breakdown of fatty acids into energy,[1] and many people find that they quickly lose weight through ketosis, especially body fat. Following this extreme sort of diet plan is therapeutic for epilepsy patients, but dieters have adopted it as a means to lose weight, even touting its other health benefits. Given the many anecdotes available on the internet, it might be easy to conclude that this is a healthy way of eating. Sure enough, many people can seem healthier by eating this way for a short time. But it's also important to remember that this is an extremely restrictive way of eating that is nearly impossible to sustain. As a result, the rebound weight gain and other negative health outcomes are profound unless people also change the foundation for their eating patterns. Long term, the ketogenic diet can be an unhealthy choice if it isn't medically necessary and especially if it isn't paired with behavioral and spiritual changes. This is because the metabolic state required during the ketogenic diet—called ketosis—is functionally abnormal. It is a compensatory process that the body undergoes to accommodate extreme circumstances. That is to say, the body would prefer not to be in ketosis, and given the opportunity, it will compensate for the physiologic stress caused by being in this abnormal state. The metabolic changes that take place during ketosis are a compensatory effect for an abnormal carbohydrate deficit that taxes the body.

In a physically healthy person, the body runs smoothly on a balance of protein, carbohydrates, and fats along with a variety of vitamins and minerals. We need *all* of these macronutrients because each organ in the body has unique nutrition needs.[2] The nutrient levels we each need change throughout our lives based on different factors[3] that are extremely difficult to measure apart from physiological body signals. Just as a growing baby has different nutritional requirements from an adult, men and women—active and sedentary, young and old, tall and short—also have unique needs.

For example, the healthy brain runs entirely on simple sugar—about 120 grams per day! It's estimated that while resting, the human brain accounts for up to 60 percent of all the body's carbohydrate requirements. The body has a specific mechanism for accessing this sugar in the bloodstream, called a glucose transporter. These transporters are the only way that glucose can reach the brain, and they keep everything else out—including dietary protein and fat. Studies have shown that during periods of starvation, the body does everything it can to channel glucose into the brain to keep the body alive. The one exception is that in periods of starvation, when absolutely no glucose is available, the brain can use ketones for energy (i.e., those produced in a ketogenic diet). However, ketones are not the brain's preferred source of fuel, and it only resorts to using them as a last-ditch effort to stay alive. This is clear evidence that in order to maintain a healthy metabolic state—God's original design—humans should regularly consume glucose-containing carbohydrates.

Unlike the brain, a healthy heart runs entirely on fat. Fatty acids from the diet are the main source of fuel for the heart. The human heart only consumes glucose when fat is absolutely unavailable. For this reason, among others, we need to consume fat in our diets so our hearts can function normally. While carbohydrates can be converted to fatty acids and used accordingly, we still need to consume a variety of plant- and animal-based fats to keep our hearts healthy. We likewise need carbohydrates to feed our brains, protein to sustain our muscles, and a variety of other nutrients so that our bodies can thrive. Any diet that supposes otherwise, whether for the sake of weight loss or health, is misinformed.

When God created the world and everything in it, he didn't haphazardly throw ingredients around until he found something that worked. Rather, he was specific and intentional. In Psalm 139:13–14, the Bible says that God carefully and premeditatedly knit each of us together in an amazing and miraculous way. He crafted every system, every cell, and every chemical reaction to work perfectly together for a unique purpose. There is reason behind creation, even all the way down to the biochemical function of the human metabolism. Given the preferential nutritional needs of the body's various organs as well as our current understanding that humans benefit from a variety of foods, our goal should be to eat in a way that promotes the optimal designated functions of our bodies. Dieting simply doesn't allow for this. In order to promote the functional state of our bodies that God originally designed, we should eat and enjoy an abundance of different foods and strive for balance rather than extremism. Of course, many medical conditions rightly warrant therapeutic diet modifications. But for the average healthy person, omitting entire food groups is not only emotionally exhaustive, but it pulls us away from God's design, leading to disease, shame, and self-condemnation.

This concept is also illustrated in the composition of our food. Natural food sources include the plants and livestock that grow and thrive on the earth without human intervention. Fruits, vegetables, grains, and animals all came into existence separately from humanity, and they were likewise created with unique characteristics. Tomatoes and chickens are biologically very different, but they are similar in that the food they provide to humans is complex. Whole foods from the earth do not contain just one nutrient, be it carbohydrates, protein, or vitamin C. Meat, in addition to the high-quality protein it's known for providing, contains vitamins, minerals, and fats that humans need. Likewise, peanuts offer more than just oils; they also offer fiber, protein, and other nutrients. Almost all of our natural food sources offer diversified nutrition, which is a far cry from vitamin pills, protein powders, and SlimFast meal replacement drinks. These products aren't natural foods; they are nutrient extracts created by man, not God.

Whole foods in their natural states offer so much more physiologically than just nutrients. As humans, we also need to regularly consume bacteria in our diets. If you're not familiar with probiotics, the "good bacteria" in our bodies, this might sound like a strange concept. However, researchers continue to discover that the human microbiome—the diverse populations of bacteria that live in and on our bodies—dramatically influences human health outcomes. These good bacteria come from more than just yogurt and probiotic supplements; they are also found on fresh fruits, vegetables, grains, and meat. These bacteria are essential for health because they remove toxins, improve digestion, and even produce many of the vitamins and minerals our bodies need. For example, the only source of vitamin B12 is from bacteria that live in the colons of animals. Since our own bodies aren't able to self-produce and absorb vitamin B12, we need to consume foods that naturally contain bacteria. In this case, the only natural source of this vitamin is meat from animals that also have these bacteria in their colons. People who don't eat meat or animal products need to supplement this vitamin from artificial sources—otherwise, they will suffer irreversible neurologic damage, eventually leading to death.[4] Another example is protein supplements and powders. Protein extracts such as whey protein are an excellent source of amino acids but are different from foods like meat that offer multiple nutrients, vitamins, and probiotics in a comprehensive and integrative way. There isn't anything wrong with consuming protein powder or similar products as part of a diverse and balanced diet; the point is that it's also OK to eat normal meals. We don't need to avoid certain foods for fear of negative health consequences, because God, who is looking out for us, designed them for us to eat.

Ultimately, the function of our bodies in their healthy state and the complementary composition of natural foods are a testament to the fact that God's creation is complex. A healthy and balanced diet can't be quantified by X amount of vegetables per day or by avoiding Y, and health likewise cannot be achieved through the isolated use of pills or powders. Observing this, it might be easy to resign ourselves to thinking that it's impossible to ever truly and completely understand the human body's needs. However, as we slowly grow in our understanding of the function of a healthy human body, we can praise God for his incredible design, which he created with passionate love. Knowing that he intentionally made our bodies to function in a particular way sets us free to embrace them, honor them, and care for them the way God intended: by eating intuitively.

Practice Curiosity Rather Than Condemnation

Intuitive eating gives our bodies the freedom they need to be healthy. But as with any change process, changing our attitude is easier said than done, and for this reason, we need to be especially aware of how our mindset might interfere with our progress. Specifically, an underlying attitude of negativity or condemnation toward our body signals can create problems as we learn to honor those body signals. Many times, we hold preconceived notions about how much, how often, or what we think we should be eating—ideas based on advertising, diet experience, and lies from our culture. Diet attitudes drive us to exercise when we need to rest, to choose a salad when we are hungry for a more substantial meal, or to skip dessert instead of enjoying a delicious treat because we are ashamed of our eating or our bodies. While you previously might have used these ideologies to make decisions about food, they ultimately drove a wedge through the connection between your mind and body, interrupting your God-given ability to read your own biological signals.

This pattern becomes especially problematic for my clients when they start to perceive their body signals again but, instead of embracing them, condemn themselves for them. They impose external "shouldn'ts" on themselves and subvert their bodies rather than embrace them. As you begin your own process of intuitive eating, you might find yourself tempted to do the same. Examples of this sort of dichotomy are the following:

- "I *shouldn't* be hungry for lunch; it's only 10 a.m."
- "I *shouldn't* eat what I'm craving because I didn't exercise today."
- "I *shouldn't* eat a snack; dinner is in an hour."
- "I *shouldn't* eat dessert after dinner because I ate a dessert earlier."
- "I *shouldn't* finish this sandwich because restaurant portion sizes are too big."
- "I *shouldn't* order French fries as my side dish because they have too many calories."
- "I *shouldn't* order a soda because soda is bad."
- "I *shouldn't* take a rest day because I didn't work out at all last week."
- "I *shouldn't* choose the full-fat ice cream because a low-fat option is available."

Any time we "should" on ourselves (pun intended), we exercise an attitude of condemnation rather than objective curiosity. If you notice yourself having a craving or a hunger pang that you didn't expect, try not to jump to the conclusion that the sensation is *wrong*; rather, try to better understand why you might be feeling that way. Perhaps you had a lighter meal the day before, were more active than usual, or are too warm and ice cream sounds particularly tasty. An attitude of condemnation ultimately says, "I wish my body was different," whereas an attitude of curiosity says, "God made my body, and I want to honor his design."

Whenever we don't honor that functional design, whether by extreme dieting or otherwise, we end up battling against our bodies. In our culture, warring against ourselves is often celebrated by the mantra "no pain, no gain." But pain is our bodies' way of telling us that something is wrong. Feeling light-headed, sore, fatigued, or anxious is not a sign of success; it's a red-flag warning, a stop sign. The same is true for dieting measures: when we can't stop thinking about food, our bodies are telling us we need to eat. I promise you, your body does not care that you're trying to get a "summer beach body" or lose weight for an upcoming wedding. It just wants to stay alive, and it's going to push as hard as it can to do that. Dieting fights against our normal physiology and detracts from our health before we even start making progress in the areas that led us to diet in the first place. Dieting is ultimately a battle against ourselves—a battle we will eventually lose.

Eating intuitively, the way God intended, effectively raises a white flag in the battle against our bodies. By embracing freedom in our approach to food, we ally with God in caring and providing for our bodies in the best possible way. Considering the examples from the beginning of the chapter of individuals who *don't* eat intuitively (Anna, the yo-yo dieter; Sam, the fitness guru; and Jordan, the mind*less* eater), we can clearly see how using food outside of God's intended purpose leads to a diet disaster: guilt, shame, and the feeling of being completely out of control. But when we approach eating the way God designed it—the way he *desires* for us—we heal our relationship with food, our bodies, and the one who made them. Through intuitive eating, we can cultivate lives that reflect God's grace and love, celebrating our bodies for all they were created to be.

CHAPTER SIX

Making the Decision

The Most Important Step toward Intuitive Eating

ran my first minimarathon in 2010. I was already an active person, but I knew there was a big difference between competing in a 5K race with my cross-country team and tackling 13.1 miles by myself. Unlike in high school sports, I wouldn't have a coach for this race; the training would be up to me and only me. I had no clue where to begin, so I started googling training plans for half-marathons. To my dismay, I was bombarded with hundreds of different schedules that *all said different things.* Somehow, after reading through all the tips and suggestions, I found myself even more confused. Overwhelmed, I turned off my computer and decided to revisit the matter the following day. During that time, I came to the realization that I didn't need to follow any one plan *exactly*, but I did need to start doing *something.* If instead of following a strict regimen, I simply embraced the principles of training (slowly increasing mileage, spacing out runs with cross-training and rest) and put those general ideas into practice, I'd be able to fit the training into my schedule in a way that complemented my unique and busy life. The single most important aspect of my training program was deciding to start.

The same concepts apply to the process of becoming an intuitive eater. No two lives look exactly the same, but despite different details, the same principles can be applied to all of our lives to help us make effective changes. In this chapter and throughout the remainder of the book, we're going to start exploring the practicality of making those changes, including the effects on the mind, body, and spirit. As you read, consider the implications for your own mindset, your own relationship with your body, and your own spiritual life. Even though you may struggle more in one area than in others, take the time to reflect on each principle so that you can strengthen the integrity of your food foundation moving forward.

Reframe Your Mindset

Which of the following foods is healthier: cookies or kale? If you answered "kale," you're not unlike the majority of the population. While kale certainly contains significantly higher levels of certain vitamins and minerals, making it arguably more nutritious than a cookie, it isn't necessarily healthier.

See, different foods play different roles in our lives. While one purpose of food is to provide our bodies with the building blocks they need for optimal function, this isn't the only purpose of eating. Even a kale salad is functionally different from a vitamin pill that contains all the same nutrients. The cool crunch of the salad is refreshing. The process of eating it provides an opportunity to catch up with a friend or take a break from a busy workday. A fresh chocolate chip cookie might not be cool and refreshing or help prevent anemia, but it offers something else to our life experience. It is warming and pleasurable. Maybe it allows you to reminisce with your grandma about the times you've baked together in the past or is a source of comfort after a chilly evening commute. Both food experiences are of equal importance; they're just different.

Viewing all foods as equal reflects a mindset of food neutrality, which is exactly what we will be focusing on in this chapter and referring to in the remainder of this book. But changing from a good food/bad food mentality to a food-neutral mindset isn't as easy as flipping a switch. Our views toward food start developing early in childhood as we observe how other people interact with food. We see others talk about different foods as "good" or "bad" and then we reinforce this moralistic type of thinking in the language we use for ourselves. The process of reframing our mindset toward food, therefore, involves unlearning that entire food paradigm. Only after doing so can we construct a more balanced perspective and begin approaching food in healthier ways—everything from cookies to kale. In order to facilitate that change, we need to pay extra attention to the language we use to describe food, whether in our minds or out loud. We also need to protect ourselves against contrary messages, including messages on food products themselves. Sometimes we even need to set boundaries in our person-to-person relationships so that we can create a safe space for healing in our own hearts. Let's dig a little deeper into those concepts.

1. Change the Language You Use toward Food

One of the ways our thought lives affect our relationship with food is when we view different foods in moralistic terms. Using words like *good* or *bad* around food lays the groundwork for unnecessary guilt and shame. To combat this moralistic thinking, we can choose the words we use about food more carefully, avoiding terms like *evil, sinful,* and other extreme descriptors. Truth be told, brownies are not evil. Fullness is not evil. But when we use language that suggests these things are bad, we start to feel bad for experiencing them. Using heavily negative words for benign things like dessert gives them power that they don't deserve. A brownie should not have the ability to make us feel ashamed or like failures; it is simply food and nothing more. In place of words like *bad* or *fattening* for rich foods, we can describe them in positive ways.

Try experimenting with phrases that resonate with you and compel you to respect food and its role in your life. Some that work for me include "Wow, this is such a tasty treat!" and "I'm so grateful to be enjoying food that I love." Thought patterns like these help me keep the perspective that eating desserts in excess won't honor my body, whereas enjoying them in a balanced way will. To get started, write out a list of things you appreciate about food and the eating experience and strive to use those words in your food-related conversations instead of negative terminology.

In addition to avoiding negative words for food, you can proactively use positive language for your body. Rather than choosing critical and condemning words, whether out loud or in your head, you can focus on speaking lovingly about your body and the way it looks. Even if you aren't quite in a place where you fully believe you are beautiful, you can practice using words that help you see yourself as God does. After all, practice makes progress.

The negative language we use toward food and our bodies usually comes from a desire to change, as if we can shame ourselves into taking action. But hating ourselves doesn't make us thinner, and it certainly doesn't help us take better care of ourselves. In fact, shame-filled words usually have the opposite effect. In choosing to use loving, respectful words toward our bodies, we sow seeds for loving and respectful behavior. Affirmations sometimes have a bad reputation for being cheesy or insincere, but body-positive language truly can be genuine, and it should be if it's going to have a lasting impact on our relationship with food and our bodies. Phrases like "I feel strong" or "This outfit flatters my figure" are good examples of places to start.

Remember that even as we are struggling to *love* the softer aspects of ourselves, such as those areas that wiggle and squish, we can meditate on the truth that God created those parts of us too. Our bodies aren't broken; they function the way their loving and kind creator designed them to function. Genesis 1:27 (ESV) says, "God created man in his own image, in the image of God he created him; male and female he created them." This means that even those aspects that we see as imperfect are anything but; they are reflections of the holiness and perfection of God, who designed all beauty for the divine purpose of his own glory.

So how shall we respond? When we feel the rumblings of negativity in our hearts, we can replace those harsh words with expressions of tenderness and grace, such as "God loves me right now, just as I am" or

"In his mercy, God has allowed me good health. For this, I will praise him!" When we focus on God's love and seek to derive our worth from who we are in God's eyes, we don't need to focus as much on our bodies. Finding our identity in who we are rather than what we look like or what we eat sets our minds free from enslavement to dieting. Make an effort to measure your character rather than your food. Instead of focusing your time and energy on the food you are eating, the calories you are burning, or the miles you are running, focus on how you exhibit God's love in your life. Focus on how you respond to others, on cultivating patience, on speaking with grace and gentleness, and on living a life characterized by God's love. The things we eat and drink don't determine how valuable we are; God loves us and our bodies, and we have always had immense value in his eyes.

2. Clean Out the Pantry

Another way to practice food neutrality is by cleaning out our pantries of labels and messages that clash with our values. Typically, pantry cleanses are encouraged as part of a new diet initiative in which we throw away foods that don't comply with the food rules. In this case, a pantry cleanse involves throwing out foods that don't comply with a diet-free mindset. In addition to billboard and TV advertisements, we are bombarded with messages about dieting on food labels. Products that boast about being low in fat, for example, make us feel that we should be eating a low-fat diet. The same holds true for statements like "Paleo-friendly," "low-carb," or "now with no added sugar!" All of these, at least indirectly, reinforce a dieting mentality. Celebrating certain aspects of food as superior perpetuates the idea that food and nutrient levels should be carefully manipulated.

Almost every single packaged product has promotional language, even down to the tape wrapping that holds banana bunches together. Of course, a person would need to exert an unreasonably high level of effort to avoid all of this advertising and would also have to limit the brands of bananas, cartons of strawberries, and bags of carrots they buy. But what is reasonable—and actually very healthy—is to avoid purchasing products that fall into an overtly diet-conscious category, including diet cola, fat-free mayonnaise, or gluten-free products (unless you have a medical reason, of course).

In addition to perpetuating a diet mentality, these products reinforce the idea that there is a reason to avoid the "real" version of certain foods: regular cola, full-fat mayonnaise, or wheat bread. According to current medical literature, there is no reason for an otherwise healthy individual to avoid any food in particular. None of these foods individually causes cancer, heart attacks, or other diseases. Overconsumption of them can, of course, contribute to some of these lifestyle diseases, but no single product is individually responsible. Exercising our freedom, rooted in our knowledge of God's love for us and our bodies, allows us to enjoy all foods, at least occasionally.

Also remember that many of these food products, despite being lower in fat, sugar, or whatever else as compared to their original counterparts, are often less healthy. While sugar-free soda doesn't directly contribute to a person's daily caloric intake, the artificial sweeteners still cause blood sugar fluctuations. The sweet taste triggers the digestive process even before the first sip is swallowed, which then results in the release of insulin, lowering the blood sugar and causing cravings for sugar. Research is beginning to emerge demonstrating that acesulfame potassium, saccharine, and other sweeteners are actually toxic and carcinogenic. I doubt companies would be as successful if, instead of advertising their products as being sugar-free, their labels read, "Causes sugar cravings!" or "Contains toxic chemicals!" Of course, the occasional Diet Coke isn't going to harm your health. But strict rules about soda and other foods perpetuate a dieting mindset, which is where the real danger lies.

Keep in mind that you don't need to exclude diet foods that you truly enjoy eating. Avoiding diet foods because of their nutritional composition is no different from avoiding original products for this reason. If you truly enjoy a cold glass of bubbly seltzer water after a meal or the extra crunchy texture of gluten-free pretzels, then enjoy them just as you would any other treat. Just be careful to not accidentally create rules for yourself about other beverages or snacks because they aren't sugar-free or gluten-free.

If you have been consuming diet products for any substantial period of time, it may be difficult to separate your true taste preferences from habitual inclinations. In this case, it may be helpful to experiment with avoiding all diet foods at first and evaluating how the original products make you feel. For example, I avoided meat for a long time because I thought that becoming a vegetarian would help me lose weight. I explained my avoidance to others by telling them that I simply didn't like meat. I eventually even convinced myself this was true and avoided meat for nearly two years. In my journey toward becoming an intuitive eater, I decided to take a break from vegetarianism and start eating animal products again. I was surprised to learn that I not only enjoyed beef and chicken but felt more satisfied and had more energy after meals that included animal protein. I've been eating meat daily ever since and never looked back. I had similar experiences with a number of other foods I'd previously avoided for diet reasons. I've gladly welcomed full-fat mayonnaise and cheese back into my life. (They give my sandwiches much more staying power than Miracle Whip.) At the same time, I realized I don't like Diet Coke nearly as much as I thought I did. In fact, I don't enjoy soda much at all! Maybe you'll find the same to be true when you give yourself the opportunity. The results might surprise you.

A number of different emotions might surface when you think about shifting away from diet products. These foods can create a false safety net by giving us the illusion of control over our bodies' nutrient levels or weight. You might find yourself worried about weight gain or an upset stomach. It could be helpful to write these fears out and pray through them, asking God to remind you of your innate worth and value so that you don't need to be afraid of dietary changes.

3. Set Boundaries

The more we are exposed to something, the more it can influence our thoughts, attitudes, and habits. Oftentimes, our views about body shape and size, diet patterns, or exercise routines are formed by the messages we receive from the media. Celebrities, TV shows, advertisements, and the things we see friends doing on Facebook or Instagram plant seeds that ultimately grow to shape our thinking. If we are trying to shift our thinking away from the generalized world view of dieting, continuing to consume media from sources that perpetuate these cultural obsessions can make it much more difficult.

I always recommend that patients unfollow people on Instagram, Snapchat, or Facebook who post about their diet or exercise routines or post pictures of their bodies that cause self-comparison. This can even be true about people who post lots of beautiful pictures of diet food. For example, I recently unfollowed someone who started posting beautiful pictures of Paleo desserts. I was finding myself tempted to compare my regular ice cream to their sugar-free coconut milk "ice cream," and even felt a little guilty for eating other types of sugar-sweetened foods. Honoring my personal boundaries by removing those pictures from my feed helped me ensure that my thoughts about food were in alignment with my personal values. Pictures like the ones I described can easily create feelings of inferiority that can do more harm than good to your own habits. If any social media accounts make you feel shame for not eating, exercising, or looking a certain way, remove or unfollow them.

This might not be easy if some of those users are close friends. One easy way around this on Facebook is simply to unfollow a user without removing them as a friend. On Instagram, you can mute accounts without unfollowing them. (Don't worry, the owner of the account isn't notified when you do this.) Other social networking apps don't have this feature, but if the person is a close friend, consider sharing with him or her that you are on a journey that involves tuning into what your body is telling you and learning to eat without dieting, and that means being intentional about your social media use. Your friend will likely understand that the boundary is for your own health and does not reflect your affection for them.

You can then proactively seek out accounts to follow (or blogs to read) that encourage a positive, loving, and freedom-oriented attitude toward food. Whether these accounts are explicitly Christian or not isn't necessarily important. What is important is the extent to which you are removing negative influences and replacing them with positive, health-promoting media. In Philippians 4:8, Paul encourages people to meditate on positive thoughts, which will transform their attitudes and behavior from the inside out. He encourages us to focus on what is uplifting, positive, and true rather than negative, writing, "If anything is excellent or praiseworthy—think about such things." Carefully choosing which food and body messages fill your mind can help crowd out toxic thoughts and empower you with the tools you need to directly combat them with truth.

Embrace Your "Here-and-Now" Body

As you practice using more body-positive language, you may find yourself becoming hyperaware of behaviors or habits that trigger shameful or negative body-image thoughts. Weighing ourselves or wearing ill-fitting clothing are two common examples that spark critical attitudes by drawing attention to areas of our bodies that we struggle to love. By removing the triggers of poor body image or reducing our exposure to them, we can lay the foundation for patterns of positive thinking, making it more likely that affirmations rather than criticisms will be the norm in our thoughts.

1. Throw Away Your Scale

Accepting the size and shape of our bodies (and our body weight) is imperative to being able to cultivate a healthy relationship with food.

When we fear weight gain or desire weight loss, it's impossible to view food in neutral terms. For many of my patients, knowing their body weight sparks feelings of shame because they weigh more than they would like to or more than they used to. Assigning so much power and influence to body weight creates enormous barriers to our progress in our relationship with food and our bodies. During appointments, patients often say things like "I was doing so well with learning to accept my body, and I was even finding myself liking how I looked. But then I weighed myself, and now I can't focus on anything other than that number." Stories such as these break my heart because as an outsider looking in, it's so obvious that body weight acceptance is a mind game. The more we indulge our desire to monitor our weight, the more difficult it will be for us to move forward in meaningful ways.

Throughout the process of intuitive eating, we often experience weight changes as we start to figure out how to read and respond to our body signals and settle into our own weight set point. During this process, we must give ourselves room to learn and grow—sometimes literally. As was the case with many of my patients, when I first started to eat intuitively, I gained weight. Giving myself permission to eat certain foods after nearly a decade of restriction led to a little bit of overindulgence. But over a few months, as my eating patterns normalized, I ended up losing the weight I gained and then some. Allowing my body to evolve was essential, and had I known my weight throughout this time, it would have posed an enormous barrier to my progress. In order to allow my body to find its own natural, healthy weight, I had to give up my desire to control the number on the scale.

Throwing away the scale is an important step toward recognizing that we generally have very little control over our bodies. Consider the amount of time you spend thinking about your body weight. When you weigh yourself, does the number affect your mood? Whether the number is positive or negative, most people will admit that it has a profound influence on their attitude, self-confidence, and motivation for the day. But the scale doesn't measure health. It pays no regard to muscle mass, bone density, hydration levels, or other important biological factors. It also doesn't measure stress levels, sleep patterns, or the richness of a person's spiritual life—all of which have far more influence over life expectancy than body weight does.

If completely getting rid of your scale feels too scary, it's OK to start small. Maybe put the scale in the bathroom closet and cut back to weighing yourself only once per day, once per week, or once per month. Maybe it would be helpful to put it in a box in the basement so that you can do a trial run of life without meaningless numbers. Whenever you have the urge to weigh yourself, slow down for a moment and think through the following questions:

- What am I feeling right now emotionally? Am I stressed? Lonely? Sad?
- When I see my weight, how will it affect me? Will I feel better or worse?
- What does the number mean to me?
- What does the number mean to God?

On days when you do decide to weigh yourself, remember that there isn't anything inherently bad about doing so; it is usually not helpful. Engaging in something meaningless doesn't mean you've done something bad. You don't need to feel ashamed or guilty for giving in to the urge, but remind yourself that the number itself does not reflect your value or worth as a human being. If you find yourself struggling with shame or self-condemnation, try actively combatting it with God-centered affirmations. For example, the negative thought "I weigh too much, I don't like my body, and I am ashamed" can be changed to "I feel uncomfortable with my body weight right now, but I also understand that I am in a process of change. I am learning to trust God with my body, and the result may be different from my expectations." Try saying these affirmations out loud or writing them down to form new thinking habits.

2. Keep Body Checking in Check

If you don't particularly like how you look, stop looking. The end goal is, of course, for each of us to love and respect our bodies as God does. But in the meantime, if your negative view of your body impedes your ability to make progress with food, it's time to put your appearance out of your mind by taking it out of your sight.

Body checking refers to the habit of repeatedly assessing the appearance of a body part (commonly arms, thighs, or tummy) to see if it looks larger or smaller than you would like it to. Many women seek out mirrors throughout the day for this purpose or fixate on reflective surfaces such as shop windows, dark computer screens, or shiny metal structures. I used to constantly look down at my thighs or seek out my reflection throughout the day to keep track of my appearance. I felt especially compelled toward body checking behavior as part of a comparison, wondering how my own appearance compared to the women around me. But staring at myself in the mirror didn't help me like my body more. Rather, it led me to become obsessed with details of my physique that I truly could not control, leaving me feeling out of control and ashamed.

If you find yourself body checking, whether by looking down at your body or looking at your reflection, gently remind yourself in that moment that the behavior is not helping you achieve your goals. Instead of seeking out reflective surfaces, start removing them. In the early stages of my recovery, I threw away or covered the mirrors in my apartment. Frankly, there isn't a need for a full-length mirror anyway. Realistically, we don't need to look at ourselves more than once in the morning, when we get dressed. If you're concerned about whether your outfit is appropriate, ask a family member or roommate or choose something else to wear.

You also might want to remove from sight any pictures that make it difficult for you to be kind to your body. For example, I've struggled with critical and demeaning thoughts about my appearance in photos and have spent hours scrutinizing the minute curves and contours of my body in albums. Once I realized how much of my life I'd wasted in agony over unflattering pictures, I decided that enough was enough, and I removed them from my phone. Even though some of these photos were of special and important events in my life, they brought up uncomfortable or overly critical emotions. I saved copies of these photos on my hard drive so that I would still have the memories, but they wouldn't be in my face, inspiring unnecessary criticism. I also found other ways to commemorate special occasions, like displaying my college diploma rather than a picture of myself at my college graduation.

3. Buy Clothes That Fit

One of the reasons we tend to engage in body checking is because our clothes accentuate areas of our bodies we aren't necessarily fond of. Overly tight jeans create unnecessary tummy rolls and draw attention to fleshier areas. The same is true for tight shirts, ill-fitting bras, and otherwise revealing clothes. While we shouldn't be motivated by shame in choosing our clothing (such as to hide our bodies or cover them up from embarrassment), we can exercise wisdom in buying clothes that are the appropriate size or have a flattering cut. My best friend has a different shape than I do, and the clothes that look best on her don't flatter my figure. The opposite is also true. While we sometimes like to borrow each other's cardigans or shoes, there's a reason we each own our own jeans. If your clothes don't fit you right now, invest in a few pieces of clothing that you can feel good in. An example would be one or two pairs of jeans and three to four tops. A small wardrobe like this can easily be purchased for $150 or less and is absolutely worth the avoidance of unnecessary body shame resulting from ill-fitting clothes. (It might also help to compare this modest sum to the money you may have spent on diet programs or fitness memberships in the past.) I especially encourage postpartum women to do this. After having babies, many women are frustrated that their prepregnancy clothes don't fit, but neither do their maternity clothes. Elastic waistbands and flowy tops can be a huge help during this time and can be both fashionable and comfortable.

4. Dress with Love and Respect

As with the previous tip, it can be helpful for our self-image to take the time to dress well. While we certainly don't need to wear gold jewelry, a fresh manicure, and designer shoes to look nice, unwashed hair and yesterday's makeup don't make us feel beautiful either. Taking fifteen to twenty minutes in the morning to put on flattering clothes, style our hair, and wear some nice earrings can make a world of difference in terms of how beautiful we feel. Try to identify the wardrobe practices that help you feel good about yourself. Whether that means putting on makeup, wearing certain colors or styles of clothing, styling your hair the way you love, or wearing your most comfortable pair of shoes, take care of your body in a way that demonstrates kindness and respect. These practices will be different for every woman, so take time to think about what makes you feel confident and well cared for.

In life, we tend to take care of the things we cherish. While an attitude of cherishing your body might not come easily to you, investing in your appearance may help you foster feelings of respect for your body. Of course, the goal here isn't vanity, but God calls our bodies temples. He created them, and he loves and values them. It's actually glorifying to God to honor our bodies by caring for them. We dress up for special occasions to honor the event. Even though the mundane tasks of daily life might not feel very holy, our day-to-day proceedings have merit. Therefore, meeting the occasion of God's calling on our lives isn't as casual as we often tend to regard it. It's OK to dress in a way that signals love and respect for our bodies, even on "unimportant" days of the week. We aren't vain or selfish for spending time grooming ourselves so that we can show up for the day with a sense of readiness, preparation, and honor. Getting dressed isn't the only way to express our love for ourselves, but it can be part of a routine that can help shape our attitudes for the day.

Cling to Truth

Changing our relationship with food involves addressing the underlying spiritual factors that drive us to eat in unhealthy ways. Although this section comes last, it certainly isn't least! In fact, it's the most important. The more exposure we have to God's affirming words of love for us, the more likely it is that we will internalize those words and allow them to transform our hearts. By reading the Bible, meditating on what it says, and being intentional about memorizing those truths, we are filling our minds with God's love and grace, thereby crowding out thoughts of food or the lies that tell us we aren't enough. These practices also help us learn more about who God says we are and how he calls us to live. The more knowledge we have of these topics, the better equipped we are to live them out.

1. Involve Your Community

If you are part of a church that offers Bible studies or community groups, I encourage you to seek the support of other believers as you take steps toward health and healing. While not all the women in your group will share the same perspectives about food and eating, they can pray for you, encourage you, and share in your struggle so that you'll know you aren't alone. No matter their nutrition habits, a loving group of women can reinforce truths about who God says you are, which will help protect you from the lies that drive you toward disordered eating behavior. God calls us to community, whereas shame and anxiety thrive when we are in isolation. Loneliness begets despair, and despair begets maladaptive behavior. In other words, when we are suffering, we sometimes take desperate measures that end up hurting us rather than helping us.

2. Pray

I also want to encourage you in this time to pray. *Hard.* Surrendering the idols of thinness and food obsession is a huge step to take in moving away from the world of dieting and back toward God's original design. Ask God to turn your heart toward his, to help you love the body he created for you, and to fill your mind with his love. If you find yourself stuck in a cycle of shame or self-depreciation, ask God to carry that burden for you. Practice interrupting negative thoughts with prayers of supplication and thanking him for success. In the Bible, Jesus promises that he will respond in kind to our expressions of faith. In Matthew 11:28–30, we read, "Come to me, all you who are weary and burdened, and I will give you rest. Take my yoke upon you and learn from me; for I am gentle and humble in heart, and you will find rest for your souls. For my yoke is easy, and my burden is light." When we live lives characterized by honor for God, we have a sense of freedom and lightness around food. God wants that for us so that we can live more freely for *him.* He will answer prayers offered in accordance with his will.

3. Cultivate Trust

Cultivating trust in God isn't about mustering up the faith to put the outcome of our circumstances in his hands; it's about recognizing that he already loves and cares for us. Sure, it's important to have faith that God will carry out his plans for tomorrow, but the greater challenge is to trust him with what's happening *right now.* We need to ask ourselves, "Do I believe that God can heal me—the whole me—the *real* me?" Can God heal our hearts even if our external circumstances never change?

When I first heard about Jesus, I believed the gospel and accepted it as my own. But I wasn't suddenly able to trust God with the most hurt and broken pieces of my heart. Yes, I was a Christian. Yes, I knew God loved me. But I was also afraid. In the beginning, I was too scared and vulnerable to bring him the broken pieces of my past. In the process of slowly cultivating trust, I read about Jesus's ministry and his words and started to apply those to my life. For example, I read in Mark 12:41–44 that God called me to trust him with my wealth by putting my money where my mouth was. The first time I dropped a twenty-dollar bill into the offering plate, my heart started beating so hard, I thought it was going to fall out of my chest. That single bill felt like a huge risk—I was saving for college, and to me, every penny counted. But later that day, I received a call from a college I'd applied to, saying they'd received unexpected donations for a scholarship fund and would be offering me a full-tuition grant. The twenty dollars from my college fund didn't need to be clenched with such a tight fist after all. (In case you were wondering, yes—that is a true story, and it is even more miraculous than that: three weeks and three more twenty-dollar bills later, I was offered *three more* full-tuition college scholarships.) To be clear, God's faithfulness and love aren't centered on our financial prosperity, and sometimes our acts of trust and our prayers lead to things we didn't want or don't understand. It's not an automatic exchange in which we trust God and he then promptly blesses us with the exact thing we wanted or needed. But for me, taking small steps of faith in the area of money was the launchpad for trusting God with all the other areas of my life. I regularly think back on that time of God's faithfulness and blessing as a reminder that he loves me and cares for me, even with regard to food.

Step Forward and Remind Yourself Why You Started

In the beginning stages of healing their relationships with food and their bodies, many women experience an enormous range of emotions, including everything from excitement and relief, to nervousness, to full-blown fear and anxiety. Most women who are unhappy with their bodies are likewise afraid of them changing in undesirable ways. The truth is that they might! But in seeking to cultivate freedom in our eating, the benefit isn't in achieving a certain physique but in the ability to transcend the hold of vanity and shame over our appearances. Pursuing an intuitive, attuned attitude toward food with the intention of weight loss will often result in failure. However, pursuing this type of eating with the hope of cultivating a sense of food freedom that will enable you to live more fully in God's love for you will yield success.

Of course, relinquishing the desire for a certain type of appearance is more easily said than done. Simply thinking to yourself "I should stop desiring to be thinner" doesn't help change your heart. But as you are praying through this process, you may find yourself coming to terms with the fact that you may never look like a supermodel. While embracing this reality is a *good* and important step, it also is a challenging one, and you might find yourself grieving the death of your hope to ever achieve your dream body. While this might sound strange, it's natural to experience sadness over something you've desired for so long. If you find yourself feeling low, that is OK for a little while. Allow yourself to grieve so that you can heal. In the meantime, keep reminding yourself why you started: Dieting made your life worse. *Not dieting* will make it better.

In the days of my eating disorder, I often would skip social gatherings to avoid food. When I did attend, I often was too distracted by the food to enjoy myself. Either my stomach would be grumbling from restricting my diet or it would be full and bloated from binge eating at the snack table. In any case, I would be preoccupied with the state of my tummy or worried about its appearance through my shirt. Holiday meals and dinner parties were miserable for me because I was unable to overcome my fear surrounding food and therefore unable to connect with my friends and family. This was the result of unnecessary food rules, food guilt, and ultimately, distance in my relationship with God. These toxic values prevented me from feeling free to engage with my relationships, enslaving me to my disordered eating and leading me to hate my life.

While I usually am glad *not* to think about those uncomfortable years, sometimes it's helpful to reflect on them because it reminds me how far I've come. It makes me so grateful for the healthy and clear mind I have now and reinforces my commitment to live (and eat) as God designed—with love for myself, the food I eat, and my body. The biggest difference between the person I was then and the person I am now isn't in my diet, my weight, or my exercise habits, however. The change that allowed me to learn to eat and live that way took place in my mindset and my heart. Deciding to try a new approach was the single most important piece of my healing journey. Without choosing to give up my desire to control my body through food and exercise, I never could have started on my path toward recovery. Instead, I would have kept living in an all-or-nothing mindset, buying diet foods, and obsessing over exercise. I consequently never would have allowed myself to learn to trust God with my body. I would never have realized what food freedom meant if I hadn't chosen to do the very thing that scared me most: let go.

CHAPTER SEVEN

Cultivating Awareness

Learning to Mindfully Listen to Your Body

ntuitive eating is all about listening to our bodies. If we believe that God designed us intentionally, then we can trust our own internal signals for hunger, fullness, and cravings. However, after a long history of dieting, many of us struggle to correctly interpret those signals. During initial appointments, my patients often tell me that they don't even know what hunger really feels like because they've resisted it for so long, eating according to plans and schedules instead of internal cues. As I will be discussing in this chapter, the way to begin tapping back into those internal signals is by practicing mindfulness. That word has quite a few definitions, but for this book, I'll be using it to refer to the practice of cultivating awareness of what's going on in our hearts, minds, and bodies. Essentially, mindfulness in this context translates to being fully present in any given moment, mentally as well as physically, and allowing ourselves to experience our circumstances without judgment. Our discussion will include practical ways to tune in to hunger and fullness cues, apply mindfulness in everyday activities like grocery shopping and cooking, and learn how to identify nonfood feelings that we sometimes misinterpret as hunger cues. Cultivating awareness in these areas allows us to effectively care for our physical needs, like hunger, but also our very important (and often overlooked) emotional and spiritual needs.

The three body signals we need to focus on through the process of intuitive eating are hunger, fullness, and satisfaction. As I mentioned, dieting has made it difficult for many of us to accurately identify when we're hungry and when we're full. But even for individuals who don't have a lengthy diet history, the concept of satisfaction can be completely foreign. Today, we typically view food solely as a fuel source without assigning much importance to factors like flavor and palatability—at least in the context of healthy eating. But satisfaction is one of the important roles God designed food to play in human life. So that's where we'll start. Then we'll follow up with a discussion of how satisfaction differs from fullness on a theoretical level. Finally, we'll explore the practical aspects of learning to identify hunger, fullness, and satisfaction and responding to those cues in a way that honors both our bodies and the God who made them.

Mindful Eating and Satisfaction

Most health resources—books, blogs, magazines, and the like—don't assign satisfaction much importance. In fact, the general argument often seems to be that the less pleasure we find in our food, the better, because then we'll eat less of it. But food and eating don't work like this because they weren't designed to. God created food, in part, to satisfy us. But if you've been a Christian all your life and never heard that before, don't be surprised. Most Christian resources I've seen completely miss the point when it comes to the intersection between food, faith, and satisfaction.

Like diet books and blogs, Christian resources tend to argue that the less we look to food for satisfaction, the better, because God alone should be our source of satisfaction. While it's true that God is the ultimate source of fulfillment, sometimes the way he goes about fulfilling us involves providing for our tangible needs—like through shelter, relationships, or food. Prayer does not satisfy physical hunger; eating does, and

God lovingly provides that food for us. Satisfying food is a good thing, given by God for our benefit and well-being. God's design for nourishment is to meet a specific set of needs—neither too much nor too little. Eating satisfying foods can therefore be an act of celebration and worship, honoring our bodies as well as the God who made them.

Mindful Eating: Satisfaction versus Fullness

Many of us neglect the role of satisfaction in our eating because we assume that fullness and satisfaction mean the same thing. But they're actually very different, and each has a different part to play in terms of helping us nourish our bodies. Consider this example: Have you ever eaten a large but light meal, after which your stomach was filled, but only for a short time? On the other hand, have you ever enjoyed a small but dense snack that kept your appetite at bay for multiple hours?

Fullness can be defined as a physical sensation of distention that results from the mechanical expansion of the stomach. In the body, this feeling is stimulated by the stretching of the stomach wall, like blowing up a balloon, which signals to the brain that the volume has changed. Fullness can be triggered by drinking water, eating a large meal, or even crowding by other organs (such as with pregnancy).

Satisfaction, on the other hand, is physical as well as emotional and spiritual. The sensation of dietary satiety is a hormonal signal rather than a mechanical one. The human body has a complex network of chemical communications that regulate appetite, physical hunger, and the biological drive to eat, which includes hormones like ghrelin, leptin, cholecystokinin, serotonin, and insulin. You might be familiar with some of these, possibly in a context other than appetite regulation, but this diversity speaks to the complexity of the feeling of hunger in the human body. Rather than simply resulting from a volume change, satisfaction depends on factors such as hunger level, body temperature, time of day, environmental setting, stress levels, season, mood, and more. The key difference between satiety and fullness is that satiety, not fullness, determines a person's drive to eat.

In their *Intuitive Eating Workbook*, dieticians Evelyn Tribole and Elyse Resch encourage individuals to practice identifying the physical sensations of eating with a water-drinking activity. In this exercise, a person slowly drinks two to four cups of room-temperature, noncarbonated water over the course of about five minutes. With each sip, he or she carefully pays attention to how the water feels in the mouth, during swallowing, as it moves through the esophagus, and then as it settles in the stomach. When the first signs of fullness are noticed, the person stops drinking.[1]

This exercise is extremely helpful for developing the skills we need to identify fullness and experience bodily sensations. It also serves as a useful tool in understanding the approximate volume of food needed to fill our stomachs. Furthermore, this activity demonstrates how different types of food and beverages affect appetite and satiety; likely within half an hour of completing the activity, your stomach will feel empty again! Many foods we eat function like water, meaning that they fill our bellies for a short time, but because they are low in energy, they don't keep us full or satisfied for very long.

A key example of this sort of food is vegetables. Many diet blogs compel readers to eat vegetables because they are relatively low in calories and therefore comply with restrictive diet plans. These bloggers often use comparison images of two different foods, demonstrating the large difference in volume between them for the same amount of energy. For example, they might show a picture of a single tablespoon of peanut butter having the same calorie count as an entire plate of broccoli along with a caption like "Look how much more you get to eat if you choose something low in calories! #EatMoreVegetables!" These graphics used to inspire me to eat low-calorie foods like vegetables or yogurt. But such a restricted diet created enormous health problems for me. In the beginning, eating this way caused me to lose far too much weight and become ill, and later, the lack of satisfaction in those plain foods caused me to binge eat. Those binges consisted of a lot more than just a single spoonful of peanut butter! Looking back, I know that if I had just chosen to eat the scoop of peanut butter when I was craving it instead of a plate of broccoli, I would have spared myself the stomachache from reactively eating the whole jar. When we try to substitute a food that is simply *filling* for a food that is truly *satisfying*, we often end up dealing with the fallout of such choices—whether by finding ourselves preoccupied with the original food or stuffed to the brim from overeating it. With time, I've found that the best approach to cravings is accurate identification and an appropriate response: identify when it's time to eat, identify what you truly want to eat, and then eat that food, without judgment, in the quantity required to satisfy yourself. In doing so, you might be surprised to find that you don't need the whole jar of peanut butter to feel satisfied.

When I coach my patients through this practice, they consistently report eating less food, enjoying it more, and feeling less stressed before, during, and after. There's a difference between merely "eating enough calories" for a meal or a day and actually feeling satisfied by our food choices. When we aren't satisfied, we end up thinking about food excessively. When we're thinking about food excessively, we *aren't* thinking about God's big picture, and that's why food satisfaction matters—so we can identify when it's time to eat, have a meal, give thanks, and move on with the lives for which God created us.

Mindful Hunger: Identifying When to Eat

Speaking of hunger . . .

In the simplest terms possible, it's time to eat when the body starts making hunger signals. Because we each have different energy needs given the context of our own unique lives, using hunger cues to determine what, when, and how much to eat rather than a prescriptive meal plan helps us honor our own body's needs much more effectively. However, doing so isn't always straightforward. Hunger signals vary significantly, even for the same individual, throughout a single day. Some of the following signs may seem obvious, but others might surprise you. Read through them and consider how you typically respond to these experiences:

- rumbling stomach
- gnawing sensation in the stomach
- recurring thoughts about food
- low energy or fatigue
- depressed, anxious, or irritable mood
- dizziness
- nausea
- headache
- poor attention or difficulty concentrating
- shakiness
- body aches
- sweating without exertion
- feeling cold
- difficulty taking a deep breath

If you start to notice these signs a few hours after your last meal or snack, they could be less-obvious indications of hunger. When I experience these symptoms, I mentally walk myself through the process of eating a snack. Sometimes the thought of eating seems like a relief, but sometimes it seems unpleasant. Often, simply visualizing the process of eating helps me distinguish between sleepiness, sickness, or other causes of the above symptoms. For example, I sometimes find myself wanting a snack or a sweet food because my stomach feels funny, or I keep thinking about snacks. But when I pause and think about how eating a snack in that moment would make me feel, I realize that I'm not hungry at all. Sometimes I'm bored, anxious, or just in need of a nap.

At the same time, sometimes I don't recognize I'm hungry even though I really am. Especially when I'm very nervous or agitated, my hunger manifests paradoxically as food aversion. The morning of my wedding, my anxiety was so high that I had an upset stomach. I remember someone offering to prepare a sandwich for me, but the thought of eating it made me want to vomit. An hour or so later, though, when the nausea had subsided, I realized that I did, in fact, *need* a sandwich. At the same time, I was grateful that I waited until the sandwich seemed satisfying instead of force-feeding myself when my stomach was upset, possibly making myself feel even worse.

Mindful Hunger: Identifying What to Eat

Once you've identified that you're hungry, it's time to eat something! The next question is what to eat. In many scenarios, the options are limited—such as when you're driving and only have a granola bar or when you're facing a time constraint while trying to get yourself (or the kids) out of the house in the morning. But when more time and options are available, being intentional about making satisfying choices helps us avoid the temptation to overeat. For example, a meal of plain brown rice, steamed broccoli, and poached chicken is filling and nutritious, but it's also bland. After finishing a meal like this, we might feel compelled to keep eating and eating because although our stomachs are full, we aren't truly satisfied. Evening snacking when we aren't hungry some-times results from a need for satisfaction that wasn't fulfilled from the previous meal. The ideal scenario would be choosing tasty, filling, and nutritious foods every time. That way, when we walk away from a meal, we are fully ready to put down our forks and move on to the next thing.

Making satisfying choices requires intentionality. When you're getting ready to cook, think through what you might eat and visualize eating that particular food. Ask yourself whether it sounds appealing or if you would likely still be looking for satisfaction afterward. Identify preferences such as temperature and texture differences. If a specific food doesn't come to mind, the following list of food qualities may help you identify the most satisfying choice:

- hot
- cold
- lukewarm
- creamy
- watery
- sweet
- sour
- salty
- crunchy
- soft
- smooth
- crisp
- dense
- light
- oily
- dry
- wet
- heavy

When making a food choice, also consider its sustaining power. With healthy, balanced eating, we need to ask ourselves not only "What sounds tasty right now?" but also "What will make me feel my best?" In certain situations, a longer-lasting and more nutrient-dense option is more appropriate, and other times, a light option is preferable. For example, on mornings when I have a busy day ahead of me, I often need a larger and more substantial breakfast. Something like a pastry might satisfy my palate but leave me hungry and irritable soon afterward. This doesn't always mean that a pastry is out of the question, but I might also eat a protein-rich yogurt along with it or choose something sweet but sustainable instead, like a peanut butter and jelly sandwich. The same holds true for afternoon snacks—some crisp, crunchy cucumbers might be the perfect pick-me-up on a relaxed afternoon, but busy days usually require some hummus or olives alongside the vegetables to keep hunger at bay.

Here's what gentle nutrition *doesn't* mean: Suppose you're at a morning work meeting, and they've provided coffee and donuts. You aren't ready for lunch yet, but you could go for a snack. You've heard that donuts and desserts should be avoided, so you tell yourself, "Donuts are full of sugar. If I wouldn't eat carrot sticks, I shouldn't eat anything at all. Donuts are bad, so I won't have one." As a result, you might move through the rest of your day totally distracted by thoughts of the donut. This is a problem on its own, but then in the evening, you might be craving sugar because you denied yourself the donut at your morning meeting, and you might end up binge eating a whole box of Girl Scout cookies. Good nutrition doesn't mean that we need to avoid treats we enjoy or restrict them to certain times of the day. Instead, it means that we need to think about how those foods will make us feel and then use that to inform our choices. If you're ready for a snack and your protein-packed lunch is in an hour, go for the donut! If it's the middle of the afternoon and you have three projects and spin class to get through before dinner, maybe it's a better idea to eat something with staying power like trail mix and enjoy the donut another time. Or you might go for the donut but eat a piece of string cheese and some tomatoes along with it to power through your afternoon. You also might choose a donut, take a few bites, and then realize you were more interested in the idea of the donut than the donut itself. In these situations, there's no shame in saving the rest for later or even throwing it away. There are a number of wise choices to make, but any decision motivated by fear, shame, or bad science will probably backfire.

We also can use our awareness of personal preferences and somatic sensations to inform our meal choices. Here's an example from my own life: I'm not really a potato person. I don't like them mashed, I don't like them French fried (unless they're covered in parmesan and truffle oil), and I really am not a fan of foil-wrapped, oven-baked spuds. I realize I am in the minority in this, since my entire family thinks I'm crazy. But the truth of the matter is that there are about a million other things I'd rather eat than potatoes in any given moment. Instead, I usually go for bread if it's being served or just forgo the starchy sides and instead take a cookie from the dessert table for my source of carbohydrates at that meal. This might raise a few questions for you, including the following:

1 Aren't potatoes less processed than bread?
2 Isn't it better to eat potatoes rather than cookies, since cookies have added sugar?
3 Isn't the *best* option to forgo the carbs altogether and eat more salad?

My answers to those questions are as follows:

1 Sure, maybe, but who cares?
2 Absolutely not, because I was going to eat a cookie anyway.
3 No, because then I'll have a sugar crash later, get *hangry*, snap at my husband, and eat a cookie anyway because I'm hypoglycemic and about to pass out.

With intuitive eating, we have the freedom to forgo food options even if they're available. We also have the freedom to choose the options we like best within a given food category even if others might turn their noses up at them. We are all called to utilize wisdom in our food choices, deciding to eat *something* because it's better than eating *nothing* but also being mindful not to eat simply because food is available. In general, nutrition is a complement to our food choices, not an overarching authority. It's intended to inform rather than dictate our eating. Below are a few of the current guidelines from the Academy of Nutrition and Dietetics regarding nutrition-informed eating practices:

Focus on Variety

- Choose a variety of foods from all the food groups to get the nutrients your body needs. Fruits and vegetables can be fresh, frozen or canned.
- Eat more dark green vegetables such as leafy greens and broccoli and orange vegetables including carrots and sweet potatoes.
- Vary your protein choices with more fish, beans and lentils.
- Aim for at least 3 ounces of whole-grain cereals, breads, crackers, rice or pasta every day.
- Think nutrient-rich rather than "good" or "bad" foods. The majority of your food choices should be packed with vitamins, minerals, fiber and other nutrients.[2]

In general, a balanced diet is characterized by lots of fresh foods, with variety, in adequate amounts. Most disease processes are perpetuated by insufficient nutrition. In other words, not getting enough vitamins, minerals, and calories from the foods we eat can make us sick. Including fruits, vegetables, proteins, fat, and carbohydrates in all our meals and snacks is a good idea. While this isn't always possible due to taste preferences, time constraints, or other reasons, if at the end of the day on most days you've consumed around five servings each of fresh vegetables, fruit, protein-containing foods, fats, and carbohydrates, you're probably receiving an optimal nutrient balance. If you include something fun at a few meals each day, you're probably feeding your taste buds pretty well too, which is equally important.

We also should pay special attention to the underlying thought processes that influence our food choices. Many times, we can convince ourselves that we have certain food preferences when they really are external "rules" or "shoulds" that we've applied to the situation without the consent of our hunger signals. An example is choosing a salad for lunch out of obligation after a heavy breakfast at a brunch café because we feel guilty for eating rich food earlier. In many cases, this is a normal and expected preference (the body self-regulates this way to balance energy and nutrient needs), but a number of times, I've been surprised by how truly hungry I am only a few hours after a large meal. It can be nerve-racking at times to submit to our body signals, especially when we have a long-standing practice of ignoring and subduing them. While it's definitely a practice that takes time, it's also necessary to honor *all* of these signals, even if they scare us or don't fit into our plans. If we are going to learn to trust our bodies, we need to honor them every single time. If you struggle with this, remind yourself that God made you perfectly and gave you internal cues for a reason. Respecting those cues honors your body and the way it was made.

To practice becoming aware of your own body's signals, take some time to think through your own experience of hunger and fullness. Rate these qualities on a scale of 1 to 10 before and after eating and then think about the quality of fullness and satiety afterward. Keep in mind that *fullness* refers to the physical sensation of your stomach expanding from the volume of food, whereas *satiation* is the absence of the desire to continue eating, which depends on types of foods eaten rather than simply the amount. Fullness can feel pleasant or unpleasant at different times, such as in reference to exercise, work responsibilities, or leisure. Considering these factors can also help you to be proactive in your meal schedule. An hour or two after you finish eating, reevaluate your hunger and satiety level and think about them in reference to what you ate at that last meal or snack. The following questions can help you get started:

- How much food did you consume?
- How long did the food keep you full?
- Was this appropriate for your daily activities?
- Would you change anything about what or how much you ate?
- If so, what would you change?

Remember that learning to read your body signals is a process that takes time and practice. If you have spent years dieting or eating without mindful awareness, don't expect to master this skill overnight. If you find yourself too hungry or too full after a meal, that's OK! These are excellent learning opportunities to help you understand your body better and empower you to make more educated choices in the future.

Try this experiment: Choose a meal next week where you will give eating your full and undivided attention. Put your phone away, turn off the TV, sit down with your plate (and your family if you live with them or roommates if you have them), and then just eat. Be fully present with your food, tasting and appreciating all it has to offer. How does the taste change after the first bite? After the third? How does the food feel in your stomach? How long does it take you to recognize that you've had enough? You can even engage others in this process if you're not eating alone. Comment on the deliciousness of the food or other aspects you like about it. It doesn't need to be a long and involved discussion, but you can encourage others by inviting them to share in your pleasure.

Practice checking in with yourself like this throughout your meals and snacks. Be intentional about choosing foods that will satisfy your cravings, ranging from main dishes to sides, from vegetables to desserts. Allow yourself to stop eating when you're satisfied and to get seconds if you sense that you need to eat more. Eat for satisfaction, and give thanks to God for his provision.

Mindfulness at the Table

Whenever possible, don't sit down to a meal when you are ravenous. If you find yourself getting hungry around thirty to sixty minutes before dinner, have a small snack. A little pick-me-up likely won't kill your appetite. Rather, it will enhance it. Urgently shoveling food into your mouth does not allow you to be slow and present at your meal and often leads to overeating. Enjoying a few bites of an appetizer, a couple of crackers, or a small piece of cheese can be enough to tame intense hunger and allow you to enjoy what the meal itself has to offer.

Before you start eating, take the time to give thanks for the meal. Giving thanks is a special opportunity to connect with God and embrace the very spiritual nature of eating. If you find yourself praying out of mindless habit, repeating the same words day after day, it may be helpful to intentionally switch up your script, invite someone else to lead the prayer, or even read a verse of scripture over the meal as a blessing. The purpose of mealtime prayers isn't to check an item off a list; it's to set the stage for truly engaging with all the elements of the eating experience, especially the spiritual ones.

When you start eating, bring all your senses to the meal. Before you take a bite, take note of the colors and other visual characteristics of the food. As you bring the first forkful closer, pause. What does it smell like? Is it a familiar smell? Does it trigger any specific memories? (Interestingly, smell is one of our most powerful memory triggers!) Also take note of the textures, how the food feels in your mouth, the temperature, and the individual flavors. How does the taste change between the first bite and the last bite? Does it improve or become dull?

In order to get the most flavor out of a meal, take smaller bites and savor them. As a child, did you ever crunch a piece of hard candy? The flavor experience is much shorter lived than when you let it slowly dissolve in your mouth. Since flavor—not just volume—satisfies us during the eating experience, we can allow the food to better fulfill us when we actually taste every morsel we swallow. Taking small sips of a beverage is another way to satisfy our senses. "Chugging" a coffee or a cola is a sure way to trigger caffeine jitters or a sugar crash, whereas slow sipping allows us to enjoy those treats with a much smaller portion. It may also be helpful to set down your glass or your fork between sips or bites to discuss your sensory experience with your tablemates as though you were enjoying art. Comment on what you appreciate about the food, and start mealtime conversations by drawing attention to the dining experience you are sharing together.

Give eating your full attention. Turn off your devices. Leave your phone in another room. Take a few deep breaths to clear your mind and decompress before you start eating. Distractions detract from our relationship with food, just as they detract from our relationships with other people. When it's time to eat, eat. When it's time to work, work. When it's time to play, play. Create boundaries around meals to protect that time and the people you are sharing it with.

Exercising Mindfulness at the Grocery Store, in the Kitchen, and Beyond

The process of mindful eating begins long before we bring a fork to our mouths. We can exercise mindful awareness throughout the process of purchasing food, cooking it, and praying over it too.

1. Mindfulness at the Grocery Store

For many, grocery shopping is a mind*less* activity—ingredients and food products are tossed into the cart based on labels, convenience, or sheer impulse. But by slowing down and checking in with the items we put into our carts, we can add value to the eating experience down the line. When we shop with intention, our eating follows suit. When you're at the grocery store, consider the appealing qualities of foods you put in your cart. Take care to select fresh, unharmed produce. If it is more visually pleasing, you are more likely to eat it later! It's easy to let food go to waste if it seems unappetizing.

Also consider the unappealing qualities of food. Are you purchasing something because you feel as though you should, even though it isn't something you enjoy? Many individuals do this with certain health food products like protein powders or vegetables they don't like. I promise, if you don't like protein shakes, countless other protein options are both convenient and satisfying, like hard-boiled eggs, string cheese, bean dips, trail mix, or yogurt. Perhaps you simply need a new recipe, or maybe the food isn't something you like at all. If you despise the texture of cauliflower, don't buy it. Never mind if Pinterest is overrun with cauliflower rice recipes; hundreds of other vegetables are waiting and ready to be eaten that will please your palate far more. In choosing foods according to our individual preferences, we can create an internal incentive to consume fresh, healthy meals. Following the same idea, if cupcakes are on sale but you don't actually like cupcakes that much, leave them. Purchase foods that you know you and your family truly enjoy eating. Food should be both nourishing and tasty, not simply a consequence of convenience. While we certainly should respect our budgets, cheap isn't a good enough reason to put something in the cart. Throwing away uneaten or expired food is the same as throwing away money. Likewise, eating food just because it's there is also wasteful and not good for your mind or your body.

Reflect on the health benefits and the role of the food in your life. Contrary to most diet advice, "I like it" actually is a good enough reason to buy something. Or maybe it's a food your spouse or your child likes, so eating it can become a shared experience with that special person. This note is particularly important for diet and health products. Many times, we purchase certain items because we have been told they are superior to their conventional counterparts (e.g., light ice cream, granola bars with added protein, whole wheat bread). While some of these might be healthful foods, eating them in excess or to replace other foods is instead an unhealthy choice (such as drinking a Diet Coke instead of eating a balanced meal). Think about how you use that food item. If your behavior with that food honors your body, buy it. If it doesn't, evaluate whether you should continue to purchase it.

Exercise your freedom in grocery shopping. Nobody is standing over your shoulder telling you what you should or shouldn't buy. It is *your prerogative* whether you buy cookies or kale—or neither or both. An empowering exercise may be to purchase a box of sugary cereal you enjoyed from your childhood even though you know it isn't the most nutritious choice and revel in the saccharine nostalgia. Likewise, you could exercise your power to try a new vegetable that you've been curious about even if it isn't part of your usual weeknight routine. Trying out new recipes takes courage, but living in food freedom is worth it.

2. Mindfulness and Food Integrity

Another way we can exercise selectivity in our food choices is by observing the integrity of what we eat. There really is something to be said for homemade food. Don't get me wrong; I love me some Chick-Fil-A and have learned my lesson the hard way that store-bought Oreos are better than the DIY variety. However, as a general rule, Grandma's gourmet is more satisfying than takeout. Part of the reason probably has to do with nostalgia, and part of it probably comes from the fact that when we work hard for something, such as by cooking it ourselves, we tend to appreciate it more. But there are also biological reasons that home-cooked meals are particularly delicious: freshly prepared food has higher levels of flavor components, contains fewer fillers, and offers more nutrition. The components of food that provide flavor (taste and aroma) are volatile. This means that they dissipate when we leave them sitting around too long. It's also why leftovers sometimes taste like the fridge and freezer-burned food is bland. Food companies try to combat this by adding some of these flavor components back in (i.e., "natural and artificial flavors"), but they don't quite have the same effect. These flavor components can also be destroyed through high-pressure and high-temperature cooking processes, which are often required to make food shelf-stable.

Just as the aspects of food that impart flavor are susceptible to the forces of heat, light, and time, many of the nutritious components of food can likewise be damaged. You might have heard that monounsaturated fats, or omega-3s, are healthy oils. This is definitely true, and we should consume foods containing these oils regularly. However, they are also very fragile. Monounsaturated oils can't sit on a shelf very long before going rancid, so most processed snacks are made with other oils that are more stable instead. Therefore, if we only consume these more processed products and crowd out fresher food, the likelihood that we will eat enough monounsaturated fats decreases significantly. While omega-6 oils or saturated fats aren't unhealthy in their own right (we need them too), we can compromise our health through unbalanced nutrition if we forgo opportunities to eat omega-3s. Monounsaturated oils are just one example of why it's generally a good idea to give ourselves as many opportunities as possible to consume a variety of fresh food through home cooking.

I want to reiterate that eating shelf-stable snacks is not necessarily an unhealthy practice. Chips Ahoy! cookies are not *bad*, and neither are those who eat them. However, it's important to recognize that a home-baked chocolate chip cookie naturally contains more vitamins and minerals along with a wider variety of other nutrients because the ingredients used are fresher. Highly refined oil used in commercially prepared cookies contains just that—*oil*—whereas fresh butter from the grocery store used in Grandma's famous recipe contains oils our bodies need along with fat-soluble vitamins and minerals. In my opinion, homemade cookies are also way more delicious. The same holds true for other types of food. Canned green beans are a tasty snack, but freshly steamed green beans have more vitamins and generally are yummier. If you're going to take the time to sit down for a meal, why not try to make the most of the experience in terms of nutritional quality and flavor? Taking the time to fully enjoy our meals helps us garner a sense of satisfaction from them, and investing time into their preparation can also benefit our physical health.

3. Mindfulness in the Kitchen

With busy schedules and multiple avenues demanding our time, cooking can often feel more stressful than it's worth. (Hello, fast food!) While home cooking usually can provide more nutrition, it offers more than just vitamins and minerals. Cooking at home, just like grocery shopping, allows another opportunity to engage with the process of eating before the food reaches our stomachs. Cooking at home forces us to slow down and create space in our hectic lives for eating. In order to learn to read our bodily signals, we need to put in the time required to practice mindfulness skills, and the kitchen is a great place to do so.

When you're cooking, appreciate the amount of work that goes into meal preparation. When it comes time to eat, serving yourself a moderate portion is easier when you realize the money and time that went into preparing the meal. It may be helpful to reflect on the process of growing the food too. A fifteen-minute trip to the grocery store is the result of multiple months, considering the time it took to plant, tend, and harvest crops. (Apple trees can take as many as seven years to mature enough to even be able to bear fruit!) Expressing awe over the intentionality and care poured into God's creation helps us cultivate an attitude of reverence when eating. This reverence helps fuel honor and respect toward both the food and our bodies.

While you are cooking, do a taste test. If the recipe could benefit from more seasoning or the omission of an ingredient you're not a fan of, take the opportunity to improve your eating experience. Appreciate the complexity of flavor combinations and how a certain spice or vegetable totally changes a dish's character. Admire details such as fresh herbs, the pleasant texture of slow-roasted meat, and the satisfying bite of perfectly steamed broccoli. Allow the food to engage all five of your senses.

During cooking, also consider how to make the food more visually appealing. While something can taste delicious even without the most glamorous of presentations, careful plating, garnishes, and intentional arrangement add satisfaction to the experience of eating. When meals offer more than just fuel, we are fed in more ways than one. Consider baking, for example. Taking the time to beautifully decorate cupcakes yields a more gratifying dessert experience. I find that they even taste better when I take the time to pipe fresh buttercream and garnish them with candy pearls rather than just haphazardly smearing the icing over the top.

4. Mindfulness through Prayer

As children of God, we are invited to worship him in everything we do, including through eating and drinking. Meals aren't usually thought of as an act of worship, but in the Old Testament, food was given as an offering to God. We can offer our meals to God today too. We simply need to set the intention.

Praying before meals is the perfect way to set the stage to connect with God. When we do this, we can give thanks for God's provision, invite him into our conversation, and express admiration and awe for the miracle of the human body. Have you ever considered how truly amazing the processes of digestion and metabolism are? Only a sovereign God can design seven billion unique creatures that each can convert a bowl of salad into skin, hair, and nails.

View mealtimes as an act of self-care. Our bodies are put through quite a bit of stress throughout the day, and it's important to supply them with the nutrients they need to repair and regenerate themselves. Being intentional about honoring our bodies with food can help us make healthy choices. God designed our bodies, so we are honoring him when we care for his creation through nutrition.

Think about the food you eat as the energy you need to show love to God and others. In order to create, worship, and engage in ministry, we need to fuel ourselves. Eating sustains our bodies and, by extension, empowers everything else we do in life. If you are feeling sluggish and slow or aren't receiving proper nutrition, your mood and energy will be compromised. Be intentional about nourishing your body so that you can pour out love into the lives of others too!

Overall, mindfulness is a skill that must be learned. It requires practice and patience, but every single person is capable of eating mindfully. It may seem awkward or uncomfortable at first, but with time, it will enhance the eating experience and open your eyes to the many spiritual aspects of dining.

Cultivating Awareness of Nonfood Feelings

If we're going to eat mindfully, we also need to learn to accurately identify what we are feeling—whether hunger, exhaustion, sadness, or something else. We've already discussed some of the different ways that hunger can manifest in our bodies, and it's important to build skill in identifying those sensations. However, it's also important to learn to properly identify and respond to the numerous *other* feelings we may experience over the course of a day. This isn't necessarily to prevent us from responding by eating, per se; sometimes eating can be an appropriate way to find comfort or boost our energy even if we don't have a grumbling stomach. (Think Grandma's chicken noodle soup.) However, the best way to address our feelings is to identify them correctly, determine the cause, and then respond to that cause rather than ignoring our feelings or numbing them away by skipping meals or overeating. The longer we ignore feelings, the more likely those feelings will compound and cause problems in our lives—and not just problems with food. Unaddressed feelings affect our relationships, our work, our spiritual health, and every other aspect of our lives.

Diving into the details of emotional self-care is beyond the scope of this book, but I bring it up because it's a very important consideration in each of our lives. Many of us turn to food for help in circumstances in which it can't actually help us, and this isn't the best way to care for ourselves in those moments. But focusing only on our interactions with food isn't going to get to the root of the problem either. If we neglect to address the underlying causes—the things that trigger us to use food outside of its intended purpose—we will continue to struggle. By cultivating awareness of our emotions and how they ebb and flow throughout the hours, days, and months, we can start taking steps toward caring for our emotional and spiritual needs more effectively. Try as we may, desserts and potato chips can't cure loneliness. They can't provide us with friendship and love or lift us out of a pattern of depression. In these instances, we must take the time to pray and reflect on the condition of our hearts or perhaps talk through our situation with a trained professional. Being able to accurately identify the underlying cause of our distress is vital for moving forward. If we are lonely, we need people; if we are in a stressful work environment, we may need a new job; if we are depressed, we may need to seek out treatment. While we *do* need food, we are also *more than food*. Humans are complex beings made up of more than just the energy it takes to keep our bodies going.

One way you can practice emotional and spiritual self-care is to keep a journal of your needs along with tangible ways to meet those needs. For example, if you find yourself frequently feeling lonely in the evenings, consider calling a friend, video chatting with your mom, playing a board game with your spouse, or inviting someone over to hang out. Things that *don't* work very well for meeting this need include eating snacks when you're not hungry, spending long hours on social media to see pictures of other people having fun without you, or ruminating about old conversations that have upset you. In the same way, watching TV or going out for a walk is not an appropriate way to respond to hunger pangs, even if we don't feel it's a reasonable time to eat. Identify body signals accurately and respond in kind.

As you work through the steps of identifying your internal cues for hunger, fullness, and satisfaction and practice self-care in terms of your emotional and spiritual needs, keep in mind that doing so is a lifelong process. Our lives are dynamic, and our experiences in our bodies reflect that. In this season, you might grow accustomed to certain predictable manifestations of hunger and fullness or certain patterns of emotions, but don't be surprised if those patterns change in a few months or years. Life will take twists and turns, and the more grace you can show yourself throughout the process, the easier it is going to be. Don't give up in moments of unsteadiness—keep your focus on God, who is steadfast.

CHAPTER EIGHT

Building a Foundation for Food Freedom

Focus on Adequacy, Variety, and Balance

When I first started learning to eat intuitively, I struggled with the daily differences in my hunger and cravings. As soon as I finally felt comfortable eating breakfast again, for example, I'd find myself hungry soon after. This frustrated me, and I started to question myself. *If I was satisfied by this meal combination yesterday, why wasn't it working today?* For a while, I resisted those ebbs and flows of hunger, but I'd end up ravenous by lunchtime if I didn't let myself have the morning snack my body was telling me it needed. All the while, my anxiety skyrocketed, and I found myself preoccupied with food-related thoughts, just as I had been while dieting. These rules that I'd created for myself about the number and frequency of my meals and snacks were holding me back from truly being able to live in food freedom. In order to move past them, I needed to give myself unconditional permission to eat. Only then was I able to learn to trust my body, find freedom from obsessive thoughts, and make peace with the woman God created me to be.

Learning to mindfully identify hunger and fullness cues, cravings, and taste preferences is only one piece of the intuitive eating puzzle. Especially for those of us breaking free from a dieting background, we need to take steps to systematically dismantle the food rules we previously used to decide what, when, and how much to eat. These rules can include anything from restrictions about types of foods, timing of meals, number of calories or fat grams, or anything else. Although this process is extremely individualized given that each person has a unique food history, the same broad principles of adequacy and variety can be applied. I start my patients on a loosely structured schedule for meals and snacks to make sure they're eating enough in terms of frequency and quantity. Once that foundation is in place, we have a steady framework to work within for breaking food rules, redeeming forbidden foods, and truly embracing food freedom.

How Food Rules Cause Problems

In a dieting context, we classify foods as "allowed" or "disallowed" (i.e., we make food rules), and then we harness every last bit of willpower to avoid breaking those food rules. When we compromise those boundaries, we feel shame, guilt, and frustration with our bodies for not behaving how we'd like them to. We then usually harness this guilt to try to drive ourselves toward compliance with the diet rules but only end up pushing ourselves further into the cycle of guilt and shame. This is extremely common with binge eating behavior. As was true in my own experience as well as in the stories I hear from my patients, food rules create restrictions, and the restrictions lead to binges. But when we remove the rules and restrictions, we allow room for satisfaction and joy in eating, and the urge to overeat evaporates.

I mentioned earlier that I used to eat a very limited diet throughout the day, consisting of little more than vegetables and yogurt, but then I would end up binge eating things like cookies, granola bars, chips, and more. In my dieting, I had created strict rules against these types of high-carb, high-fat, prepackaged foods and did my best to avoid eating them. The mental and emotional strain from such restrictions paired with the enormous energy deficit I'd accrue throughout the day left me completely exhausted by the evening, when I'd throw caution to the wind and eat as many sweets and snacks as I could get my hands on. I'd end up completely weighed down from a combination of physical fullness and unbearable shame. Overcome with guilt, the next morning I'd vow to do better, strengthening my resolve to stick to my clean eating plan. But willpower wasn't the problem; the restrictions were. Once I removed the food rules and started trusting my body to tell me what to eat, I finally interrupted the restrict/binge/guilt cycle at its beginning. Permitting ourselves to eat according to our body signals is essential in avoiding the compulsion to frantically *over*eat.

Allowing ourselves to eat does not mean we should indulge every whim to put something in our mouths. The key concept in the process of eating intuitively is that of giving ourselves unconditional permission to eat *with mindful awareness*. This involves a little more than simply eating when we are hungry and stopping when we are full. I think most of us would agree that simply giving ourselves unconditional permission to eat . . . and eat . . . and eat . . . would not be healthy. Rather, this would likely be binge behavior, which does not honor our bodies. What eating with awareness *does* mean, however, is that we permit ourselves to eat when we feel hungry even if we don't think it's reasonable to be hungry again so soon after the previous meal or snack. It also means we allow ourselves to enjoy the foods we are craving even if they have a bad reputation in the health food world.

Start with a Structured Framework

In a clinical setting, the idea of going from strict food rules to eating without any type of schedule or structure seems overwhelming to patients. It's too much too fast. Transitioning into intuitive eating is a process, and a lot of learning takes place along the way. In order to facilitate that process, I work with my patients to create a loose framework for meals and snacks to use as a guideline for getting started. (I still observe these guidelines for myself today.) Having a structured framework helps ensure that we are eating enough food in terms of both frequency and quantity so that our nutritional needs can be met. Nutritional adequacy is important not only for physical health but also for spiritual well-being. When we aren't nourishing our bodies, we don't have the energy we need to care for ourselves or others or to invest in a relationship with God. Each day, we have a far greater purpose than to eat and drink. If an unbalanced way of eating interferes with our ability to accept ourselves, care for others, and engage with life, we need to do something differently. We need to eat early enough and often enough so that our hunger doesn't get out of hand and distract us from the fact that food is just one small part of life.

1. The 3-2-1 Framework

I typically structure my eating schedule (as I likewise advise my patients) with what I call the 3-2-1 framework: each day, aim to include three meals, two snacks, and one dessert. Of course, this is flexible—some days you might be hungrier, and some days you might sleep in right up until lunchtime. But for the most part, this eating pattern supplies our bodies with a steady stream of energy while preventing us from getting so hungry that we feel compelled to overeat. As a general rule of thumb, we should eat every two to three hours. While your body's own preferences may differ somewhat, two or three hours between meals and snacks is a good place to start. You may find that you aren't hungry between meals, but giving yourself permission to eat a snack helps remove subconscious restrictions you may not even realize you have. For individuals who have been eating in unbalanced ways for so long that they are completely unable to perceive the sensation of hunger, intentionally following a more structured eating plan helps restore those hunger and fullness cues. If you can relate to that experience, more structure may be better for you in the beginning. But even if you don't feel particularly disconnected from your hunger and fullness cues, you still need to eat regularly. Erratic and unpredictable eating patterns trigger maladaptive behavior and can amplify the body's stress responses.

On the other hand, some of my clients are familiar with their hunger but afraid of it. Instead of allowing themselves to snack between meals, they resist the urge to eat until they can't anymore, resulting in a binge. When we skip snacks, our hunger can become out of control, leading us to eat far past the point of fullness. For many, this feeling is then followed by guilt and shame. Many people try to avoid snacks because they think these will prompt them to eat more food than they would otherwise. Sure, this is true for mindless eating uninformed by *awareness*, but in general, we eat far more at meals if we let our hunger get out of control.

I usually arrive home from work around 5:30 p.m. For the most part, my husband and I can get dinner ready within thirty to forty-five minutes, and we generally sit down to eat by 6:30 p.m. But sometimes by the time I finish work, I find myself hungry enough to eat dinner as early as 5:00 p.m. While I *could* wait another hour and a half before eating, I've learned that if I *do* wait that long, I am usually irritable, low energy, and positively famished by the time dinner is ready. I don't make the best dinner company in those instances and usually greet my husband by saying, "Hi, I'm starving. Talk to you after dinner." Then I proceed to frantically shovel food into my mouth until I'm overly full and exhausted from the stress of such strong hunger pangs. I've found that eating a snack, even as late as 5:00 p.m., is not going to spoil my appetite. Something as simple as a piece of string cheese or a handful of pretzels (or an appetizer if I'm at a restaurant) helps keep overwhelming hunger at bay so that I don't find myself in an almost intoxicated state. In these instances, eating a snack before dinner helps me enjoy my meal even more. Stuffing food into our mouths because we're extremely hungry doesn't allow us to taste and enjoy what we're eating. But if our hunger is at a more reasonable level, we're able to eat slowly enough to garner pleasure from eating and feel satisfied by our meals.

Contrary to what most diets advertise, snacking is not a bad thing. Rather, snacks help us keep a steady flow of energy throughout the day, thereby preventing blood sugar swings, irritable moods, and overeating. While certain snack choices might provide lasting energy and nutrition better than others, there's no reason to avoid your favorite chips, crackers, or whatever else—even at snack time. Exercising wisdom in nutrition sometimes means eating processed snack foods, and sometimes it doesn't. Sometimes it even means doing both! When I need a snack, I often find myself fantasizing about Cheez-Its or Oreos, but I know these foods won't keep me going for very long like snacks with more protein and fiber would. I approach these situations by pairing "quick energy" foods like crackers or cookies with something that will slow down the digestion process and provide fuel for my body more slowly over time. For example, I'll pair an Oreo or two with a cup of yogurt or eat string cheese and some celery with a handful of Cheez-Its. Chemically speaking, the carbohydrates available in Oreos or Cheez-Its aren't very different from those found in fruit or whole-grain bread. However, they might have very different effects in terms of my satisfaction, and if I don't choose something satisfying, I'll keep eating past fullness.

It takes some time to get to know your body's own patterns of hunger and fullness. But once you follow a steady pattern of regularly scheduled meals and snacks for a month or two, you will likely start to feel hungry around the same times each day and have an accurate idea of how much you need to eat to satisfy your hunger long enough to reach your next meal or snack. Throughout this process, it's extremely important to make sure that you regularly supply your body with energy so that you can become reacquainted with what healthy and normal hunger and fullness signals feel like.

2. Balance and Variety via Gentle Nutrition

In addition to being regular, it's important that our meals are balanced, meaning that they contain sources of protein, fiber, fat, and carbohydrates. (In an ideal world, we would balance our snacks like this too, but doing so isn't always practical—sometimes we have limited access to snack foods.) In the framework of intuitive eating, we refer to this as *gentle nutrition*. While I definitely don't advocate counting macronutrients (or counting anything, for that matter), paying attention to these nutritional balances is important for keeping our hunger and blood sugar levels stable. Protein and fat help keep us full and satisfied, allowing us to receive a steady supply of energy after meals rather than creating energy "highs" and "lows." It's also important to include a source of carbohydrates at every meal too, though. Meals that are too low in carbs can cause blood sugar to drop later in the day and lead to intense cravings and overeating. At the same time, avoiding light foods like fruits and vegetables altogether can make us feel lethargic and uncomfortable.

If all that sounds like too much to keep track of without dieting, don't worry. A helpful tool I use with my clients to help them gently observe nutrition guidelines is the plating method. This involves dividing the plate into quarters and filling up each sector with a portion of fruit, vegetables, carbohydrate, and protein and then incorporating fats and oils throughout. An example is a scoop of pasta (carbohydrate) with meat sauce (protein and fat), a side of salad with dressing (vegetable and fat), and some cinnamon apple sauce (fruit). Since meals aren't always built from individual components like that, I also encourage clients to just make sure that among the foods they eat, each macronutrient category (carbohydrates, protein, fiber, and fat) is fulfilled. An example is a burrito bowl with beans and rice (protein, fiber, and carbohydrate), cheese (fat and protein), roasted corn and tomatoes (fiber), and grilled chicken (protein). A general rule of thumb for snacks is to include at least two macronutrients to help ensure adequate energy and variety throughout the day. These methods can be used to build meals at home, at a friend's home, or out at a restaurant. They are both flexible and intuitive—perfect for a free and balanced lifestyle.

One of my patients came to me for help because he was having a hard time finding ways to fit balanced eating habits into his demanding schedule. He was seldom home, so he ate almost every meal out at restaurants. He almost always chose foods like burgers and French fries because he found those foods to be most satisfying. In a session together, we discussed the importance of eating vegetables for his health, and I suggested he order a vegetable side dish instead of potatoes or bread, as his entrée typically already offered him enough carbohydrates to satisfy and energize him. His response was not uncommon: "The vegetables don't taste as good as fries to me, though. There's no point in eating something if it doesn't taste good." Of course, this patient wasn't denying the importance of vegetables but rather expressing the fact that the steamed broccoli at Culver's just doesn't taste as good as onion rings.

With intuitive eating, we make food decisions based on satisfaction but also incorporate knowledge of how our bodies feel. A healthy diet must include vegetables in some capacity, and the current recommendations from the CDC encourage eaters to fill half their plates with produce.[1] (This is the basis of the plating methods described above.) While a dieting mentality might caution us against flavorful toppings like sauces or preparation methods that add calories or fat to vegetables, the intuitive eating perspective compels us to make those fruits and veggies taste as delicious as possible so that we can be satisfied by foods that provide our bodies with the nutrients they need. Taste and nutrition do not need to be mutually exclusive; they can and should complement each other.

Using palatability and nutrition in complementary ways with food means looking to amplify the satisfaction factor of nutritious foods like vegetables. Spinach blends into smoothies with almost no trace of taste, carrots and celery make wonderful additions to soups or sauces, and I personally have yet to find *anything* that doesn't taste good after being sautéed in butter. Adding a high-calorie or "nutrient-void" topping to a food does not negate the beneficial components of that food. For example, adding ranch dressing to carrots doesn't make the carrots unhealthy or suddenly void of fiber. Buttering a sweet potato doesn't wipe away the vitamins it naturally contains or make the potato "unclean." Dipping strawberries in chocolate doesn't take away from the vitamin C, magnesium, or folate they provide. Sweetened dried cranberries are still cranberries; broccoli in cheese sauce is still broccoli; zucchini fries are still zucchini. Are some of these variations higher in calories, fat, or sugar than their raw, fresh-from-the-farm counterparts? Yes. But they're also probably more filling and more satisfying and provide longer staying power. No matter what you hear about the health effects of dairy, gluten, or sugar, adding cheese to broccoli, breading and frying eggplant, or dipping brussels sprouts in aioli does not make those vegetables unhealthy. *Not* eating vegetables is an unhealthy practice. Seasoning vegetables to improve palatability is actually a health-promoting behavior because it increases the likelihood that we will eat these foods! When we prepare vegetables to be truly delicious, we don't need to overeat other foods in order to feel satisfied.

Another way to improve the satisfaction factor of bland but nutrient-dense foods is to hide them inside of more palatable recipes. Highly palatable foods are foods that universally taste good, usually because they are high in salt, sugar, or fat. These foods have a bad reputation in the diet world because mindless eaters tend to overconsume them. (Think whole buckets of popcorn at the movie theater.) Of course, we understand through the science and practice of intuitive eating that we don't need to actively restrict or monitor these foods in order to use them in a balanced way. However, in the ideal nutrition scenario, the majority of what we eat offers quality nutrition to fuel our bodies and honor our health. We can maximize the quality of our eating patterns by adding more nutritious ingredients to tried-and-true recipes. For example, my favorite chili recipe includes numerous rich ingredients: a whole block of cream cheese, a whole block of cheddar cheese, plus the obligatory sour cream topping. Eating a small bowl of this chili satisfies my taste buds but doesn't necessarily fill me up. However, if I were to eat a bowl large enough to fill my stomach, I'd feel sick! I also would have finished my meal without allowing myself to include other types of foods, like vegetables.

Instead of dampening the mood of the fiesta with a side dish of carrots, I add extra vegetables to my chili to amp up the nutrition, lighten the load, and help me feel my best while still enjoying a tasty and filling dinner. Pureed cauliflower and shredded zucchini are virtually tasteless on their own, and I don't notice a difference when I mix them into a boiling pot of spicy, cheesy chili. The only apparent difference is how I feel after eating it, and it's definitely a positive difference! I do the same thing with other recipes too. When my husband and I cook, we almost always double the amount of vegetables called for in recipes and amp up the spices too. (Sometimes the extra vegetables dilute the flavor.) By hiding the vegetables in the main dish, we eliminate the temptation to forgo them in favor of a second helping of something else.

No matter your place along the eating freedom journey, I strongly caution you against following any eating framework that doesn't include fun foods and/or fun food preparation methods. Sustainable eating patterns are those we could follow every day for the rest of our lives. The likelihood that a person could eliminate pleasurable foods from their diets for the rest of their lives without falling into binge eating behavior is very slim. Make an effort to be proactive about including foods you enjoy in your diet, including desserts. Not only is pleasurable eating a gift from God, but it's not going to harm your health if you respect your cravings with a sense of awareness.

3. Meal Planning

Another way to ensure adequacy and variety in our diets is by planning ahead at the beginning of the week to make sure we have access to the food we need to nourish our bodies well. Meal planning is a popular practice lately, but many social media feeds endorse it for diet control. This is a key example of how a practice or behavior can be healthy and proactive but also diet-centric and detrimental to health. I advocate for meal planning because it helps us ensure that we have access to balanced, satisfying meals and snacks throughout the day, every day. Whether at work or at home, on the go or resting, it's vital to eat well. This is extremely important for maintaining a healthy relationship with food and promoting long-term physical health. If we don't believe we will be able to eat when we need to eat, we may end up overeating out of self-protection. The purpose of meal planning should *not* be to

- distract you from fun food opportunities,
- enable adherence to a strict diet regime, or
- provide a means for counting calories, macros, points, or anything else.

Meal planning is supposed to free you, not enslave you. If you find yourself not wanting the lunch you packed on a given day, save it for the next. If you have been craving a donut all week, get a donut. If it's your coworker's birthday, share a piece of cake with them. Engage in behaviors that free you up to lead a healthy life—mentally, physically, and spiritually.

I approach meal planning from an intuitive eating context by focusing on my favorite meals of the week and building other meals around those. For me, that means starting with dinner. By planning out four tasty and satisfying dinners to cook at home and writing out a grocery list, I can usually recombine those ingredients to make enough meals and snacks for the whole week, with a few additions. Here's an example:

- Four dinners in a given week might include beef pot roast, chicken stir-fry, spaghetti (with meatballs, broccoli, and garlic bread), and a frozen pizza with salad. Leftovers can be eaten for additional dinners, or you can eat out at a restaurant.
- Lunches that week can include leftover salad from the pizza night topped with chicken (from the stir-fry), meatball sandwiches, beef sandwiches, or leftovers. I also often keep peanut butter, lunch meat, and bread on hand for easy, last-minute lunch ideas.
- Snacks can include extra raw veggies that weren't in the stir-fry or pot roast (bell peppers, carrots, pea pods, broccoli) along with hummus. I also recommend buying three to four types of fruit and two to three snack foods (like pretzels, granola bars, or nuts).
- Breakfast is usually pretty basic on weekdays, made from staples like oatmeal, eggs and toast, yogurt with granola, and some fruit and coffee. Whatever you typically like to eat for breakfast, buy at least four days' worth of two different breakfast options.

Supplement with fruit, which can double as a snack. Likewise, yogurt and granola make great snack options, as do hard-boiled eggs.

- Desserts are generally straightforward too. Each week, buy one or two different types of desserts, like a pint of ice cream and brownie mix, a package of Oreos and a take-and-bake pie, or ingredients for your favorite cookie recipe.

Again, the purpose of meal planning is to help ensure you have access to satisfying and nourishing food regularly throughout the day. From meals to snacks, even down to dessert, thinking ahead a little can help you make sure you don't run out of staple ingredients before your next grocery trip. When we don't have food on hand that we enjoy eating, we often end up overeating because we aren't fully satisfied or undereating for the same reason. Both lead to problems down the road, and meal planning helps avoid them.

As you begin transitioning out of a diet context, the structure given by the 3-2-1 eating schedule, the plating method, and meal planning act as a safety net. Like dieting, they offer a sense of predictability, but unlike dieting, they are flexible, individualized, and designed to empower you to honor your body instead of fighting against it. In order to put the other principles of intuitive eating into place (like food freedom, for example), we need to have a solid foundation, and the structure outlined in this chapter provides exactly that. Now that the groundwork is laid, we're ready to start incorporating those principles of flexibility and intuition by restoring food freedom.

CHAPTER NINE

Redeeming the Forbidden Fruit

A Systematic Approach to Breaking Food Rules

With an established, predictable pattern of meals and snacks, we develop a mutual sense of trust with our bodies. When our bodies know they will be fed regularly, hunger signals become predictable and steady. When we grow accustomed to those hunger and fullness patterns, branching out to include different types of foods feels much more manageable. With a loosely structured eating framework, substituting "forbidden" foods for diet-friendly foods is much easier and more straightforward, and it helps prevent us from feeling overwhelmed when we start intentionally breaking our old food rules.

Rules about what, when, and how much to eat are a huge roadblock to intuitive eating. Whether we are dieting or not, cravings exist. But having rules against the foods we crave prevents us from truly honoring our bodies. Simply following a predictable eating schedule isn't enough; even diets have those. To become intuitive eaters, we also need to eat freely within that framework, enjoying our favorite foods without guilt and shame. One of the essential components of growth in the ability to identify and respond appropriately to cravings is believing—and acting on the belief—that all foods are created equal. I've already said this, and I'll say it again: cookies and kale are both important parts of life. While they may serve different purposes for us on a nutritional level, they both play an integral part in satisfying us. The media has been making a big deal about processed foods lately, and advertisers use language that elicits fear, bias, judgment, and moralistic thinking about food. For example, added sugar has been described as dangerous, toxic, deadly, and the source of diabetes, obesity, and poor performance in school. No wonder so many people are afraid of it!

Sugar-sweetened foods tend to be at the center of the majority of my patients' food rules. We previously discussed the false claims about sugar being addictive, but countless other accusations are thrown around in conversations about sugar. Because sugar is such a huge topic in diet-focused media, I want to delve a little deeper into this subject in particular. Breaking food rules is a lot easier when we know that they don't hold any true merit. Let's revisit the science.

Sugar is a chemical consisting of tiny molecules linked together. It provides us with quick energy by driving chemical reactions in our cells. If we link enough of these energy molecules together, we call the substance starch. When we only link one or two together, we call it sugar. Likewise, if we take a long chain of these molecules (i.e., starch) and break it back down into its individual components, such as through digestion, they revert to sugars, and our bodies then use them as such. In the process of digestion, long-chain carbohydrates such as those found in bread or potatoes are slowly broken down, gradually releasing sugars. This is why complex carbohydrates are considered a source of long-term energy, whereas sugars are thought of as quick energy.

When we eat a food that is relatively higher in simple sugar, we experience a sugar rush. Biologically, our cells are exposed to high levels of sugar, make a lot of energy, and use it quickly. After the energy is used up and the high wears off, we may experience what is called a sugar crash. Most of us have experienced this, particularly on Halloween nights after devouring candy for hours. Repeated bouts of sugar rushes and crashes throughout our lives can be problematic. This unbalanced and extreme way of eating taxes our digestive organs and can lead to disease. However, if we eat a sugary food along with other foods that take longer to digest, such as those high in protein, fat, and fiber, the sugar isn't released into our bloodstream as quickly, we avoid the sugar highs and lows, and we protect our organs. In other words, eating sugar in an unbalanced way is unhealthy, and this is the source of the radical claims that sugar is toxic or dangerous. However, eating sugary foods in a balanced way, the way that God intended, is healthy, normal, natural, and safe. Just like drinking too much water can drown us from the inside out, sugar can be dangerous if used *incorrectly*.

The same is true for the other aspects of food that have acquired bad reputations over the years. From high fat to dietary cholesterol to gluten to food additives, almost no part of the human diet is immune to scrutiny. Indulging in this scrutiny breeds a preoccupation with food, and such obsessions harm us physically, emotionally, and spiritually. Food is just food, and it is a morally benign aspect of life when we keep it in its proper place. Therefore, in order to keep things in perspective, we need to stop viewing certain foods as good or bad. When I started experimenting with intuitive eating, I had my own fair share of reservations about food neutrality. I had spent so many years believing otherwise, but when I started taking action in my own life by intentionally breaking my food rules, the proof was in the pudding: nothing bad happened. Instead, my relationship with food, with my body, and even with God all improved dramatically. It was 100 percent worth every bit of discomfort I endured in the process, and I guarantee it will be worth it for you too. Let's dive in.

1. Figure Out What Your Forbidden Foods Are

Food rules are highly individual. A person who has been following a low-carb diet likely has a very different list of forbidden foods than someone who has been following a vegan diet. In order to make peace with food and give yourself unconditional permission to eat, you need to identify your personal roadblocks in your own life. Start by making a list of the most obvious forbidden foods you can think of, such as the foods that weren't allowed on your most recent diet plan, or rules that immediately come to mind about the timing of meals and snacks, amounts of food, or certain ingredients. But don't stop at the obvious rules, because the hidden ones often cause problems down the line. To figure out the sneakier food rules, I often encourage clients to take a trip to the grocery store. The purpose of these trips isn't to pick up the items they usually buy but rather to make note of the things they *don't* typically buy—because their food rules have forbidden them from doing so. I encourage you to take a trip like this to your own grocery store too.

When I completed this exercise for myself, I was surprised by how many food rules were lingering in the back of my mind that I didn't even realize I still had. As a kid, I loved Oreo cookies. They were my favorite snack to buy from vending machines when my grandpa gave me his spare change. When I'd ride my bike to Dairy Queen with friends, I always ordered a mint Blizzard with *triple* Oreos. I was all about the cookies 'n' cream life, at least until food rules came into the picture. Throughout my years of dieting, I avoided prepackaged sweets and snacks strictly enough that I pretty much forgot about Oreos entirely. They were so off-limits for me that it did not even occur to me to walk down the cookie aisle at the grocery store. But when I slowly started becoming an intuitive eater, I had an aha moment one day at the supermarket. As I wheeled my cart through the store, I suddenly realized I could incorporate about fifteen additional aisles of items into my diet that I had been completely ignoring, including some of my favorite foods. I systematically worked my way up and down those aisles over the course of a few years, reintroducing childhood favorites like Goldfish crackers and butter pecan ice cream into my life (and yes, Oreos too). Breaking my rules about prepackaged sweets and snacks gave me the freedom to eat them when I'm craving them without panicking afterward. Today, eating a few Oreos with my lunch or after dinner doesn't feel like a big deal; it's just part of life.

2. Systematically Breaking Food Rules

Another major food rule I had in my days of disordered eating was against ice cream. In fact, I was afraid of it. It almost feels silly to say that now, as it conjures up the image of a giant bowl of soft-serve stomping through a Warhol-esque cartoon town, sending terrified children running in all directions. But of course, a fantasy dessert monster isn't what scared me about ice cream. My fear came from the belief that going out for a sundae would change my body for the worse. I was afraid of losing control, afraid of disliking my appearance, afraid of becoming unlovable, and afraid the ice cream would lead to all those things. I was scared that if I allowed myself to eat ice cream, I'd eat, and eat, and eat and never stop. But that's not what happened. Instead, I slowly grew tired of it, and the urge to binge eat entire tubs completely disappeared.

Giving myself permission to eat ice cream whenever I wanted broke its power over me. Eating ice cream with regularity allowed me to learn how it affected my body. In eating ice cream, I learned that I liked the taste of certain flavors, but others weren't as satisfying. I learned that if I ate three scoops, I started to feel queasy, but if I ate one or two, I felt pretty good. I learned that if I ate only ice cream for breakfast, I'd be hungry again in a few hours, but if I ate it as a snack or before bed, I felt more balanced. Eating ice cream in the winter helped me realize that being chilled to the bone was unpleasant enough to sway my desire for it, whereas a hot summer day makes it taste like the most delicious and refreshing treat ever. Eating ice cream helped me learn that a daily dessert isn't what causes me to gain weight, develop high cholesterol, or get diabetes—binge eating does. The fundamental foundation I needed in order to start healing my relationship with ice cream was giving myself unconditional permission to eat it.

When I say I gave myself unconditional permission to eat ice cream, I really mean it. The summer I first started surrendering my food struggles, I spent about three weeks eating ice cream multiple times per day. I ate it with breakfast, as a morning snack, with my lunch, and before bed. I experimented with ice cream bars, freshly made gelato, the grocery store tubs, and the hand-dipped gourmet style. I ate soft-serve, triple-churned, low-fat, and creamy custard. Slowly over those weeks, ice cream stopped tasting as good to me. Eventually, I didn't want it at all anymore, except maybe once every few days. Then the craving only came once every few weeks. At first, I would be uneasy about the cravings, afraid that they would never subside. But as they grew less and less frequent, I began to trust both my body and the process of cultivating attunement. Today, I am completely secure in my relationship with ice cream, and I fully believe that when I allow myself to eat it, my body will tell me when to stop. Usually, I'm satisfied after just one small scoop after dinner (though I occasionally steal a bite of my husband's too). I also know that I don't prefer soft-serve or reduced-fat varieties or anything that's too *vanilla*. I'm a chocolate girl, through and through, and I know how to use that self-awareness to make a satisfying dessert choice that feels good in my body.

When I work on systematically breaking food rules with my clients, I teach them to treat their food rules the way I treated ice cream. Within the 3-2-1 framework, we plan to incorporate the forbidden food into every meal and snack until it loses its allure and just becomes a regular option for a snack, side dish, or dessert. In doing so, we view the forbidden food—whatever it may be—in terms of its macronutrient constituents and then plug it into the framework wherever it belongs. With one client, it was bread and butter (carb + fat); for another, it was chicken wings (fat + protein); and for a handful, it was ice cream (carb + fat) just like me. I went through this exact same process with every food on my forbidden foods list: Oreos, peanut butter, cereal, and even whole milk. Look back over your own list of food rules and forbidden foods. Which food will you start systematically incorporating into your life first?

3. Cheat Days: The Wrong Way to Go about Breaking Your Food Rules

In order to break food rules and truly heal from a dieting mindset, we need to eat forbidden foods every day. If we don't interact with those foods as a part of normal, everyday life, they will continue to haunt us. Treating them as special or attempting to restrict them in any way, such as to certain days of the week, gets in the way of our ability to cultivate trust in our bodies. One of the common practices in the fitness and dieting world today is the idea of a "cheat day," in which individuals follow a strict dieting protocol on most days but then allow themselves to eat with abandon for one day every week or two. Essentially, these days are planned binge eating episodes, and people typically eat two or three times as much food as they might normally eat, made up of different ingredients than usual, often to the point of feeling sick. The idea behind this practice is that a cheat day keeps dieters from feeling deprived, making the diet feel easier. But the benefits of cheat days are purely theoretical. They don't manage cravings effectively, as demonstrated by repeated episodes of binge eating week after week. As you might expect, this type of eating creates more problems than it promises to solve. Binge eating sugary foods is extremely challenging for the digestive system. It's so much healthier to space out sweets and snacks as part of a balanced meal schedule throughout the course of a week than to eat an excessive amount of them over the course of only a single day.

Similarly, planned splurges or cheat days foster unhealthy thinking patterns throughout the week and encourage a phenomenon in which a person overeats in anticipation of future restriction. In this situation, a dieter typically has permitted herself to eat unlimited amounts of food for one evening with the resolve to start over anew the next day, resuming the strict diet and limiting herself once again. The thought pattern usually goes something like this: "Tomorrow, I won't be allowed to eat this. I'd better get my fill now, because this is my only chance." This is how a woman is led to eat an entire jar of peanut butter in a single sitting, whereas she might ordinarily eat that same jar over multiple weeks if she were to eat in a balanced way.

Planned splurges create an attitude of impulsiveness. We don't need to eat something just because it's our "cheat day," especially if it isn't something we aren't craving. Intuitive eaters know they can enjoy their favorite foods every day of the week, not just on special occasions reserved for indulgence. They also know they don't need to eat something just because it's available. If they're at a restaurant and craving a salad, they don't feel the compulsion to order a pizza to honor the special occasion. Likewise, they don't feel the need to finish the food on their plates at any given meal, because they know they can enjoy that same food again the next day if they so desire.

One afternoon, I saw a colleague eating pad thai at her desk. While I'm not usually a fan of Asian noodle dishes, seeing her twirling the rice pasta with chopsticks made me suddenly crave pad thai with overwhelming intensity. When I got home that evening, I told my husband that I wanted to go out for Thai food. He happily obliged, as he is always a fan of international cuisine, and we went out to order the largest possible portion of chicken pad thai, extra spicy. It was amazingly delicious and exactly what I was craving. However, since it was an enormous plate of food, I had a very full takeout box to bring home with me. I enthused about the delicious noodles the rest of the night and started talking about it again first thing in the morning. I even reheated the pad thai for breakfast, fully enjoying every spicy twirl of noodles alongside a hefty side dish of well-deserved teasing from my husband. I smelled like fish sauce and garlic all morning, but I didn't care. I was satisfied and happy, and my husband still wanted to kiss me despite my bad breath.

Pad thai is not typically seen as a health food, and most dieters avoid such dishes due to the high fat, carbohydrate, and salt content. In my days of disordered eating, I definitely didn't allow myself to indulge in such foods, usually because I was afraid of losing control around them. Pasta was a food I'd find myself regularly overeating. It tasted so good that I thought I couldn't stop. But today, as a happy balanced eater, pad thai and other pasta dishes don't scare me because I know I'm not powerless over them. Instead of trying to suppress my cravings, I embrace them—even at breakfast. Doing so allows me to enjoy treats moderately, whereas avoiding my favorite foods begets fear. I don't just save sweets, treats, and special dishes for once in a while; I include them in my life regularly and am healthier because of it.

Sometimes we fall into the cheat-day attitude or plan splurges surrounding special events or holidays. Most celebrations involve food in some capacity, and the meals served are often richer and more decadent than usual. Naturally, we might feel drawn to eat more than on ordinary occasions. Viewing certain foods as more special or exciting than others can lead us to overeat them because we've allowed them to have undue power over us. One of the ways to combat this in the beginning stages of freedom eating is by intentionally eating rich and delicious foods like pad thai with regularity.

Rich foods have a bad reputation because they are associated with health problems. The standard American diet is notorious for high proportions of cheeseburgers, pizza, and French fries, and because of the poor health of many Americans, we view these foods as responsible. But they aren't actually causative—at least not directly. Americans suffer nutrition-related health problems not because of cheeseburgers but because of the frequency with which they consume such foods. Eating cheeseburgers all the time crowds out the opportunity to eat other important foods, such as vegetables. A diet consisting of only cheeseburgers or only pad thai does not lead to good health outcomes. This is obvious. But if avoiding your favorite foods leads you to binge eat them whenever you finally cave in to your cravings, as I had experienced with ice cream, you probably should be eating them more often.

4. Mind over Matter? Maybe Not

One of the ways I help myself build trust in my body and avoid overeating is by keeping a variety of desserts in my house at all times. I have a dedicated shelf in our pantry that has two or three types of chocolate, a few types of fruity candy, and a couple different types of shelf-stable cookies. I keep ice cream in the freezer most of the time too. This way, when I have a craving, I know I can fulfill it. Sometimes simply having that knowledge is enough to satisfy me—no eating involved! My husband often teases me about my hoard of sweets, but having them available helps me keep them from usurping power over my life. Attempting to reserve sweets for "special occasions" not only led me to overeat my favorite foods, but I'd end up binge eating foods I didn't even like. Giving myself permission allows me to make satisfying choices that keep my cravings from getting out of control. Instead of my making a big deal about sugar by creating rules around it, I accept that sugary foods are just a part of my life. When I'm craving something sweet, I choose a food I truly love and then move on. Likewise, when I'm not craving sweets, I don't feel compelled to mindlessly munch on them. This is a completely opposite experience from when I put forth enormous amounts of energy trying to avoid eating sweets but ended up binge eating them anyway.

Even if you are very controlled about your approach to sweets and snacks, the mental effort required to avoid those foods ends up giving them more power than they deserve. Fearing the result of eating a food, whatever the reason may be, is essentially becoming enslaved to it. When we are afraid of a certain food, we assign it value, influence, and control over our lives that it is not worthy of having. While *fear* may seem too strong a word, mere aversion is a form of submission too. If we avoid certain foods because we don't like the taste, we are the ones in control. If we avoid a food because we don't like the idea of what it might do to us, the food is in control. Food and our bodies are not our enemies; *fear* is our enemy, and rather than leading us to self-care, it leads us into a dieting disaster. The only way to overcome the fear of food is by eating it.

Sometimes we try to manipulate our attitudes toward certain foods by convincing ourselves we dislike them, for example, and it isn't usually successful. If someone were to say, "Don't think about a pink elephant," most people wouldn't be able to get that image out of their minds. The same holds true for forbidden foods. The moment we tell ourselves we shouldn't indulge becomes the moment we can't stop thinking about indulging. Even if we try to convince ourselves that we don't "like" the food, it still holds a certain draw.

Another of the more common reasons for food rules has to do with managing health conditions rather than weight loss. Many women I have worked with struggle with gastrointestinal symptoms such as stomach cramps, constipation, diarrhea, and gas. While the diagnosis for these symptoms is very common (usually irritable bowel syndrome [IBS]), there aren't many effective prescription drugs available to provide relief. Patients continue to grapple with their debilitating condition, taking over-the-counter pills and following the FODMAP diet (a restrictive diet commonly recommended by physicians). Interestingly, one of the most common underlying causes of IBS is anxiety. It doesn't matter what is causing the anxiety; the stress response manifests physically in the same uncomfortable way. Of those looking for nutritional support for their IBS, more times than I can count, the problem is not food but the stress and anxiety surrounding food. For these patients, their disordered eating behavior (and other stressors) causes mental agony, which takes a physical toll on their bodies. Their emotional and spiritual struggles transform into a physical one, manifesting as IBS. In an effort to ease their symptoms, they further manipulate their diets, cut out foods, and change their exercise regimens. But doing so ends up perpetuating their stress, worsening their symptoms, and worsening the problem. My prescription for them is behavioral coaching through the practice of intuitive eating, not the diet they expected.

I see patients with IBS symptoms very frequently in practice. Because I work in an integrative setting (alongside health care providers from other backgrounds, such as acupuncture, massage, and nutrition), the majority of the patients who come to our clinic are interested in natural, noninvasive treatment options such as diet and lifestyle modifications. Many have already tried different interventions before they even come to my office, such as eliminating gluten or dairy from their diets. Sometimes, these attempts involve whittling down their diets to just a few foods in an attempt to manage their symptoms. One patient had reduced her diet to nothing more than apples, bananas, and protein shakes. She started by removing dairy from her diet, which seemed to help at first, but then her symptoms returned. So she started avoiding gluten, then anything fried, then certain types of vegetables, and so on. Although the increasingly restrictive diet wasn't helping her symptoms, she continued it because she thought it was the right thing to do. She had no idea that her restrictive diet was harming her rather than helping her. This sounds like an extreme case, and it is, but situations like these aren't uncommon. Even more common is when patients expect *me* to tell them to restrict their diets like this. The sighs of relief I hear when I tell my patients to eat *more* rather than less honestly make me so sad. Restricting our diets to the point that they make us stressed, sick, and exhausted is *not* what I would call a holistically healthy lifestyle, and it's not the type of relationship with food that honors and supports our bodies.

CHAPTER TEN

Guarding Your Heart

(against the Temptation to Diet)

Self-defense is pretty much common sense. We don't need to take martial arts classes to understand that protecting ourselves from harm and taking precautions in risky situations are generally good things to do. We wear seat belts in the car, helmets on our bikes, and harnesses when we go rock climbing. We lock our doors when we leave the house, wear sunscreen at the beach, and when we cook chicken, we make sure the internal temperature reaches 165 degrees—just in case. As humans, there are certain areas in which we are inherently vulnerable, so taking a few precautions in life not only helps us survive but can also help us thrive. Likewise, in areas in which we've previously been harmed, we tend to be especially careful. I worked as a nanny for a semester when I was in college, and I still remember the excruciating pain I felt when I bent over to pick up a toddler and ended up wrenching my back in all the wrong ways. You'd better believe that nowadays, every time I reach down to lift something heavy, I squat low, brace my core, and lift with my legs. If there is any question that the object may be too big or cumbersome, I defer to someone else. Three minutes of convenience is just not worth the *three months* it takes to recover from a back injury.

When it comes to our eating philosophies, we also need to take a few extra steps to protect our hearts and minds with regard to our relationship with food. In the early stages of becoming an intuitive eater, the concepts of food freedom and body acceptance are new and fragile. A few bad days, a hard conversation, or even a particularly persuasive advertisement can trigger us to resort to old ways, undoing all our hard work and setting us back. While slips and lapses in recovery are nearly inevitable, the more we can avoid them, the better off we will be. In order to protect ourselves against these stumbling blocks, we often need to set strict boundaries about the types of media we consume, certain thinking patterns, and even interpersonal relationships. But before we discuss those in detail, let's take a deeper look at the importance of this sort of boundary setting.

The Biblical Basis for Boundaries

Food and drink pose an extremely difficult problem for Christians in the Western world. We are bombarded with temptations from every direction, especially the temptation to engage in diet extremes—whether indulgence or avoidance. Our social education starts from a young age, teaching us that our identity comes from our appearance and suggesting that since *we are what we eat,* we'd better not get the whole eating thing wrong. With some areas of temptation, it makes a lot more sense to cut the subject out of our lives and run in the opposite direction, but we can't do that with food. As complicated and frustrating as eating can be, we need to keep doing it—every day. This is why it's so important to set up safeguards for ourselves in this area of our lives and turn away from influences that tell us lies about the role of food. In healing our relationship with food, we can't just clean out the old ways and stop there; we need to fill the space with a new perspective of grace, honor, and compassion. Then, and most importantly, we need to protect ourselves from future temptations so that when they come, they can't penetrate our hearts.

Shortly after I became a Christian, I experienced some significant progress in the realm of my eating disorder recovery. My new faith was exciting to me, and I was blown away by the rich community I found through the church. As a brand-new Christian, I was inexperienced and more than a little ignorant. The bliss of knowing God and experiencing his freedom led me to believe that since I made the decision to follow God, all the work was done. Unfortunately, it wasn't. In my initial leap into food freedom, I neglected to realize that my past vulnerability in the area of eating would make me susceptible to falling back into my old habits in the future. When college came around and I faced some difficult life circumstances, the struggle left me weak and afraid. Having neglected to put up safeguards around myself against the temptation to indulge in harmful behaviors, I stumbled back into the grips of my eating disorder. This time when I fell, it was harder and farther than before. But thankfully, my final fall jarred me enough that I was able to fully surrender my struggle and experience new life.

As Christians, we are invited to live in truth and freedom. Allowing ourselves to return to a diet-centered approach to food is unwise, draining, and can even be harmful. Paul says it perfectly in Galatians 4:8–9: "Formerly, when you did not know God, you were slaves to those who by nature are not gods. But now that you know God—or rather are known by God—how is it that you are turning back to those weak and miserable forces? Do you wish to be enslaved by them all over again?"

Sometimes, Christians get it wrong and believe that their dieting preoccupations are in the name of the Lord. Have you ever heard it said that because our bodies are the temple of God, we should honor our bodies and keep them in excellent condition? Indeed, we read in 1 Corinthians 6:19–20, "Do you not know that your bodies are temples of the Holy Spirit, who is in you, whom you have received from God? You are not your own; you were bought at a price. Therefore honor God with your bodies." Christian dietician Kylie Mitchell writes, "Growing up, when I'd hear people reference any scripture referring to the body as a temple, I felt like I was being told that temples were beautiful so I should be striving to conform my body to the standards set by our broken world. (Become thinner. Take up less space. Eliminate dessert. Eliminate carbs.) But now I realize that a temple isn't made *to be worshipped*, it's a place to worship! When your body becomes what you are worshipping . . . it's idolatry."[1] When the Bible says that our bodies are temples, it doesn't mean that we are supposed to build, sculpt, and adorn them to be beautiful according to the standards of the world. Rather, that verse refers to the powerful truth that we were made beautiful from the very moment we were created by God. That beauty serves not as the focal point of the creation but rather as a reflection of the deeper power, honor, and glory that resides within the temple—the beauty of our hearts.

Guard against Legalistic Thinking

One of the key areas of our thought patterns to which we need to give special consideration is legalism. Legalism is the perspective that our value and worth are found in what we do rather than who we are—beloved sons and daughters of Christ. At first glance, it might not seem that diet-related thought patterns are legalistic. But if we take an honest look at the way we view ourselves and our lives, some other patterns might likely emerge. For example, what types of behaviors make you feel guilty? Of course, robbing a bank or performing some other criminal act would be a reason for guilt and shame. But what about how much you eat, the types of foods you choose, or the amount you exercise? Do you feel guilty after serving yourself a second helping of pasta or a piece of Aunt Marge's famous apple pie? Do you feel bad for sleeping past the alarm for your 6 a.m. spin class or when a woman who is thinner than you starts jogging on the neighboring elliptical at the gym? All of these negative self-perceptions come from an underlying attitude that there are moralistically superior ways to eat, exercise, and appear and that those who fall short are somehow less-than. But all this guilt stems from the lies of legalism. Gossip is sinful, lying is sinful, and murder is sinful. Eating chocolate cake isn't a sin. We are lovable, valuable, and worthy of respect because we are made by God—not because of our exercise habits or eating patterns.

A few of the more common myths and lies that people often hold today regarding the moralism of our food choices are as follows:

- Eating meat means you don't care about the environment.
- Eating dessert means you are a bad steward of your health.
- Being in a larger body and not actively pursuing weight loss means you are lazy, stupid, or gluttonous.
- People have thin bodies because they are careful eaters and diligent exercisers.
- Superfoods will make you live longer.
- Vegetarians are healthier.
- God doesn't want us to kill, so we shouldn't kill animals for food.
- I can't trust my cravings.
- I could be thinner if I had enough willpower.
- I need to be thin to be beautiful.
- If I eat processed food (i.e., "bad food"), then I am bad.
- There is something wrong with me because my body looks different than I wish it looked.

As another example, some of my patients are afraid of adopting a sense of freedom in eating because they think it means they will be "letting themselves go." By this, they mean that by eating with abandon, they will become negligent of health, wellness, and fitness and consequently succumb to illness, a drab appearance, and sloth. This is absolutely not the case! The goal of intuitive eating is to encourage people to honor their bodies by responding appropriately to their bodily signals. Neither skipping meals nor binge eating honors our bodies, and dieting is what perpetuates those practices. *Not dieting*, therefore, doesn't equal *not honoring* your body. Done correctly, freedom-based eating is the most God-honoring way to approach food. In doing so, we not only respect the creation of God (1 Corinthians 19) but can free our minds of food-related thoughts so we can see ourselves as God does (verse 20).

To protect ourselves from legalistic thinking, we need to practice identifying when we are falling into those thought patterns. Then, when we recognize them coming on, we can pause, pray, and remind ourselves of what we know is true. By meditating on God's grace and remembering how deeply we are loved, we discredit the lies of legalistic thinking patterns and return to a mindset of self-care and compassion.

Guard against Reactionary Diets

Another common trigger for relapsing into diet behavior comes from episodes of overeating that might take place as you practice breaking food rules, redeeming forbidden foods, and restoring your relationship with your body. Learning how to identify fullness and satisfaction signals takes time, and being able to identify a satisfying snack with staying power isn't a skill that develops overnight. Especially in the beginning stages of learning to eat freely and intuitively, overeating still might happen. This is normal and expected. Early in our work together, many of my patients express fear that intuitive eating isn't working for them. They find themselves overeating as they work to reintroduce some of their forbidden foods, sometimes even triggering full-on binge episodes. Naturally, this scares them, and they find themselves tempted to return to dieting to make up for the binge eating. But returning to diet behavior is actually the worst thing you can do in terms of your progress. We must take precautions not to lash out against the binge with restriction.

Many people will feel guilty and disgusted after an episode of overeating and resolve to skip the next meal, eat low-calorie foods, exercise excessively, or engage in other types of penance behavior. The guilt and shame are visceral and intense. I know that it's hard to sit in an uncomfortable space without trying to do something to alleviate that discomfort. However, those reactive patterns of restriction and self-punishment are problematic. They are part of disordered behavior, and continuing to follow them will push you further backward. Continuing to do the same thing you've always done is going to give you the same miserable results. In order to move forward again after a step backward, it's essential to push through the discomfort and keep honoring your body with regular meals, rest, and grace. In the hours or days after a time of overeating, resist the temptation to react. Instead, respond with wisdom and grace. Even if you aren't hungry, eat breakfast. Nourish your body and allow your digestive system the benefit of following a regular eating pattern. With time, the discomfort from the binge or overeating episode will subside, and you will be far less likely to overeat a second or third time if you keep eating enough and eating often. Honoring your body under God also means having the freedom to make a good choice even if it isn't what feels good in the moment.

Another thing to keep in mind is that relapsing into a time of overeating doesn't mean you have failed. These instances can be learning experiences, so use them as such. Reflect on the experience and try to identify what might have triggered the lapse. Had you been inadvertently restricting yourself in the days leading up to the overeating episode? Had you been spending time with others who were engaging in extreme eating patterns, talking about dieting, or indulging their own body dissatisfaction? Perhaps the binge occurred after a period of stress at work or at home. Maybe you were operating outside of your normal routine or you experienced a traumatic or shocking event. Learn to identify the connection between life events and your tendency to engage in unproductive eating behavior. Then use this information to inform your future self-care practices. For example, during times of stress at work, take extra time in the evenings to unwind, such as by taking a hot bath, getting a massage, or enjoying leisure activities. If you experience a difficult situation, take the time to process your emotions rather than trying to avoid them. Allow yourself to cry. Allow yourself to become angry, and shout into a pillow to relieve the stress rather than bottle it up inside. Sitting with emotions is uncomfortable, but so is sitting with the aftermath of a binge.

Transitioning away from a long-standing disordered relationship with food is not as quick as flipping a switch. It's a circuitous route, and we sometimes find ourselves reverting to maladaptive behavior at times. As I remind my clients, patience is key. Don't give up, stick it out, and try to trust the process. Intuitive eating really does deliver on its promises—something diets can never do.

Guard Your Heart by Setting Boundaries with Others

Sometimes as we are making progress in the realm of freedom eating, we come to identify legalistic attitudes in others, whether by outside observation or by the fact that others are outwardly imposing them on us. Many well-meaning friends and family members may feel that they have insider knowledge regarding the human metabolism and may share dieting anecdotes, suggest we not eat the things we are eating, encourage restrictive behavior, or even say outright cruel and offensive things to us about the things we eat, the types of exercise we choose, or the way we look. Whether these comments come from a critical and judgmental spirit or a place of love, the truth is that we don't have to internalize the attitudes of others. In fact, we have a responsibility before God to hold ourselves accountable and to foster thinking patterns that enable our freedom to lean into the truth of his love. In Colossians 2:16, we read, "Therefore do not let anyone judge you by what you eat or drink, or with regard to a religious festival, a New Moon celebration or a Sabbath day." While these friends and family members might not outright say that they think you are less *holy* because of your food choices or pants size, any degree of moralistic high ground associated with these things is, at the end of the day, legalism.

While today's culture is one of the largest influences on our collective values regarding food, body shape and size, and exercise, sometimes we face even stronger influences in our lives—our parents. Often, well-intending parents micromanage their children's eating habits by restricting certain foods, force-feeding others, and expressing expectations of exercise and activity levels. Other parents are even more controlling and critical, taunting, teasing, or even outright shaming children for gaining weight, eating sweets or snacks, or resting. For developing minds and hearts, these criticisms and shaming behaviors are often internalized and carried into adolescence and adulthood. Hypercritical or controlling parents can create deep wounds that only intensify with age and become all the more difficult to overcome once they've set in over the course of a couple decades.

As children, we can't stand up to our parents; they are our authority. Even if parents are good at listening to the hearts of their children, most kids just don't have the skills and maturity to say, "Hey, Mom, your side comments and eating restrictions are damaging my relationship with food and pointing me toward shame and self-condemnation. Leave the eating and exercise up to me, OK?" But as adults, we *do* have the power to protect ourselves, and there may come a time when it's necessary to assert boundaries regarding our food choices. While God calls us to pursue peace and protect relationships, if others in your life are speaking lies to you about your value and worth on account of your body, you are under no obligation to stand for it. Instead, you can calmly ask these family members to respect who you are and the freedom you have to exercise authority over your own body. You can even take the opportunity to share with them that you have struggled to keep food from taking over your life and that in times of dieting, you are too distracted or stressed to live a healthy, balanced life. This should be a respectable answer, but there may still be people who fail to pay you appropriate respect in this regard. If being in the presence of certain individuals in your life in food-focused situations harms your relationship with God, choose not to share meals with those people. (In situations of outright abuse, please seek professional counsel and help.) Setting boundaries doesn't need to be harsh or cruel; it can be done with kindness and wisdom. But it needs to be done; otherwise, we set ourselves up to get hurt over and over again.

In the face of undue condemnation for your food choices or exercise habits, cling to the truth of God's love for you and your body, just as you are. As we are called in Philippians 2:16, "Hold firmly to the word of life." Some will disagree, some will oppose you, and some may even hurl insults at you, but you are under no obligation to indulge thought and behavior patterns that lead you to feel guilt and shame, even if the people you love expect you to engage in them. The gospel has set you free to live in the freedom of who you are rather than live in bondage to diets, even if everyone else around you isn't following suit. Diets take away our power, allowing outside forces to dictate the way we live. Likewise, succumbing to pressures from other people to follow specific eating rules gives them power over our lives that they don't rightfully have under God. Galatians 5:1 reads, "It is for freedom that Christ has set us free. Stand firm, then, and do not let yourselves be burdened again by a yoke of slavery." Take the initiative in protecting yourself so that nothing compromises the joy and fulfillment of knowing your value in the eyes of God.

Guard against Hidden Forms of Dieting

Dieting can be defined as a rigid food plan or health paradigm that dictates what to eat, when to eat it, and how much you eat. Pretty straightforward, right?

While the folly of certain food-related behaviors may be obvious to you, others might not be so obvious. Many bits of eating advice may appear helpful or right, but they really are diet behaviors in disguise. As you move along in your journey toward becoming an intuitive eater, be mindful that many of the diet-related messages you encounter in the media might not outright seem like diet advice. In fact, they might label themselves otherwise but secretly be selling messages of food and body shame. In Matthew 7:15–16, Jesus warns us that falsehoods may masquerade as truth, but we can identify these lies by their outcomes: "Watch out for false prophets. They come to you in sheep's clothing, but inwardly they are ferocious wolves. By their fruit you will recognize them. Do people pick grapes from thornbushes, or figs from thistles?" In the realm of eating, we can likewise identify "wolf in sheep's clothing" by the promised fruit. As a reminder going forward, any eating advice that makes a radical promise, such as increased longevity, weight loss, or the ability to prevent disease, likely is (a) a lie and (b) a diet. Even if there is some truth behind the claim, it likely has been exaggerated, taken out of context (especially the context of a scientific study), and twisted to convey falsehoods. Sometimes a twisting of the truth is more difficult to spot than an outright lie, and these hidden diet messages are sometimes even more dangerous to us in the beginning stages of intuitive eating than overtly obvious ones.

Health bloggers are a particularly common source of disguised diet information—even bloggers who claim to have a nondiet message. In reading these blogs, we need to exercise extreme caution. First of all, many health bloggers aren't as healthy as they seem. In her eating disorders webinar, Nicole Hawkins (PhD, CEDS) shared results from an interesting 2014 study of "healthy living bloggers," in which 24 percent of the bloggers studied had clinical eating disorders, 33 percent had menstruation or fertility problems, 76 percent were currently on a diet or had recently dieted, and 52 percent included some form of written negative or guilt-inducing messages about food on their blogs.[2] So not only might your favorite food blogger not be as healthy as she claims to be, but she might be unintentionally influencing *you*, her reader, to engage in unhealthy behavior. Don't take everything you read at face value. The ugly truth is that most of the things you will come across on food blogs are wrong, misleading, or dangerous. The ones that are evidence-based, trustworthy, and forthcoming are much harder to come by. Don't stop questioning the authority, honesty, or ulterior motives of the things you read on the internet. In fact, it might even benefit you to avoid reading these types of health and wellness blogs for a few months (or even years) as a means of guarding your heart and mind in your healing journey.

Guard against Out-of-Context Nutrition Claims

In this book, we've discussed freedom-based eating as a paradigm that is, for all intents and purposes, universally applicable. Of course, there are obvious exceptions to the rule of "all foods fit" in cases such as allergies, for example. Someone who is allergic to peanuts absolutely, 100 percent should not include peanut butter in his or her life. That's just a bad idea. But otherwise, exercising complete food freedom is a right that every person, whether underweight, overweight, diabetic, celiac, or suffering from an autoimmune disorder, has under God. However, for some of these particular conditions, there is a sound medical reason to restrict a person's diet. As a health care provider, I recommend diet modifications to my patients on a daily basis. However, the approach in these cases is to manage a disease rather than to encourage weight loss for the sake of weight loss. I also am careful to consider the whole health of the person, including emotional, social, psychological, and spiritual factors, before I ever make such a recommendation. Most notably, I make sure that my patients have a healthy relationship with food before I ever consider prescribing a therapeutic diet for them. When considering the risks of nutrition therapy versus the benefits, recommending dietary interventions to patients with a history of, the propensity to develop, or an active eating disorder could literally be a matter of life and death. In the context of nutrition therapy, the relationship with food always, always, always has to come first.

That's also why this discussion about when diet intervention is appropriate has to come last in this book. Without laying the groundwork for establishing a healthy relationship with food, a mindset of dieting or disordered eating can easily distort this information, possibly even causing more harm. I almost didn't include it in the book at all for this very reason, as I don't have the luxury of sitting down with each and every reader to talk through the nuances on an individual level. However, nutrition therapy is such a huge part of my day-to-day life as a functional medicine physician that my clinical work might seem like a contradiction to the message of this book if I didn't address it. So here goes: nutrition therapy is appropriate when it's appropriate, and it's not when it's not. In order to discern between those two scenarios as a health care provider, I work closely with each patient in light of the following considerations.

1. Nutrition Therapy Isn't Appropriate in All Contexts

One of the conditions typically managed with nutrition is ulcerative colitis, which is an inflammatory bowel disease characterized by profuse diarrhea, bleeding, weight loss, and nutrient deficiencies. Many patients become so ill that they require hospitalization or surgical resection of the bowel. Sometimes they even lose the ability to eat altogether and end up needing to receive nutrition through a nasogastric tube. One of the ways that these patients can be helped is through physician-monitored diet modification and high-dose nutrition supplementation. Certain foods that trigger symptoms are removed, and others are added in with higher-than-normal proportions. While the diet modifications are extreme and time-consuming and need to be followed with both accuracy and consistency, the payoff is that patients can heal enough to prevent the need for a colostomy bag or feeding tube.

The psychological toll taken by the strict diet required for healing in these cases is significant. Illness is very difficult to cope with, and as with other potentially fatal conditions, the treatments themselves are taxing to every aspect of a person's life. With all medical disease interventions (such as prescription drugs, chemotherapy, and surgery), the person needs to be healthy enough to withstand the intensity of the treatment, or it will cause more harm than good. The same is true for diet modification. If a person has a long-standing history of dietary restriction and eating disorders, the likelihood that a nutrition intervention will trigger a relapse for that individual is high. Eating disorders are not a lighthearted matter—they are among the deadliest of all mental conditions. Along the same lines, if attempting to improve physical health through nutrition comes at the expense of *spiritual wellness*, in my opinion, the intervention is harming a person rather than helping them.

Nutrition and behavior expert Ellyn Satter created a model called the hierarchy of food need, in which she demonstrates how a person must have a strongly positive relationship with food before his or her diet can be manipulated without causing problems. In Satter's language, before a person can use food instrumentally, such as for a medical purpose, he or she also needs to be secure in knowing he or she will receive *enough* food, *acceptable* food, *reliable, ongoing access* to food, food that *tastes good*, and food that is *novel*.[3] While some of these food-related requirements may seem excessive, for someone with a complicated relationship with food or a history of eating disorders, research has clearly demonstrated that failure to meet these food needs can trigger severe and potentially life-threatening relapses into eating disorder behavior. Some people can make dietary changes without a problem, but other people can't. Without screening the eating behavior of my patients before suggesting a diet modification for medical reasons, I could end up contributing to their suffering instead of alleviating it.

2. Even If an Illness Can Be Managed with Diet, It Doesn't Mean the Illness Was Caused by Diet

In college, I met a pastor on a mission trip who had been diagnosed with pancreatic cancer in his twenties. After undergoing chemotherapy treatments and surgery, he became diabetic. (Without a properly functioning pancreas, the body can't produce insulin and therefore cannot properly metabolize carbohydrates.) As a diabetic man, he carefully monitors his eating and limits his carbohydrate intake to prevent complications. Avoiding sugar is one of the ways that he manages his disease, but this in no way means that sugar caused his disease.

In fact, we don't have any evidence to support the idea that eating sugar or anything else independently *causes* diabetes, cancer, heart disease, stroke, accidents, suicide, or any of the other leading causes of death in the United States. While many conditions can be treated through nutrition, especially those involving autoimmune reactions, the person's diet isn't what caused the disease, and that person likewise isn't to blame for his or her condition. I have both close friends and family members who have advanced-stage Lyme disease, which is an inflammatory bacterial infection that can last a person's entire life. The disease is transmitted by tick bites and can be difficult to diagnose in the early stages. However, if it *isn't* treated early, it can manifest as a severe and potentially life-threatening chronic disease. Aside from antibiotics right after the tick bite, the disease can't be treated with medications. Rather, the only way to manage symptoms is through nutritional support and careful monitoring by a physician. Deviations from these diet plans can allow symptoms to flare up, whereas adherence to these plans keeps the symptoms at bay. Does a "bad diet" cause Lyme disease? Absolutely not. Can dietary modification *help* Lyme disease patients? Absolutely.

3. Eating with Freedom Is Still Possible, Even with a Medical Diet

Just like a person with food allergies, individuals with evidence-based and medically supervised dietary interventions can (and should) still strive to eat intuitively. Eating with freedom involves more than just the types of foods eaten; it's a framework for eating in general, involving careful attunement to body signals and appropriate responses. Individuals allergic to wheat, for example, should still eat a varied diet filled with protein, colorful vegetables, adequate carbohydrates, plenty of fats, and fun, palatable foods. While they can't eat wheat bread due to the risk of life-threatening reactions, they can certainly choose delicious and satisfying wheat-free options. If you are following a medically necessary diet, I encourage you to still pay careful attention to your hunger, fullness, and satisfaction signals so that you can honor your body and take good care of it. If you can't eat gluten because of an allergy, that doesn't mean you can't enjoy cookies, cakes, or pasta made from gluten-free grains. At the same time, binge eating gluten-free baked goods still leads to the same physical, emotional, and spiritual consequences as binge eating wheat products, so it's important to apply the same principles of intuitive eating to a gluten-free diet as we would to one that includes gluten.

4. The Confusion of Gluten

Even outside of autoimmunity (allergies, intolerances, etc.), many people today believe that gluten-containing foods are outright unhealthy. Likewise, some people even claim that humans were never meant to eat grains. While it is true that individuals who have gluten allergies should not eat gluten-containing grains, for the vast majority of people, eating gluten is perfectly fine. Humans have been eating gluten-containing foods since the beginning of time. God provided bread as food for his people countless times throughout history. The fear-inspired aversion to gluten really is a phenomenon of the modern world. Today, thousands of people follow gluten-free diets yet receive absolutely no benefit from doing so. Gluten-free diets do not reduce disease risk in healthy individuals, and they don't lead to weight loss on their own.

Now, I want to make one thing clear: there's nothing wrong with following a gluten-free diet, even if you don't need to do so from a medical standpoint. Avoiding gluten is not necessarily harmful in its own right. However, making a restriction like this can set a person up for disordered eating behavior. As with other food rules, sometimes we can fall into the frame of mind that one food rule is all we need, and as long as we follow it, we can eat as much as we want of whatever we want. But even if all we ate was green vegetables, a diet of endless kale is not healthy. Whether following a gluten-free diet or not, we still need to check in with our body signals and honor them. Avoiding gluten won't save us from this responsibility. It also won't save us from gaining weight, as many people hope.

The notion that gluten-free diets lead to weight loss is completely unsubstantiated. Sure, if a person looked at his or her diet and removed all gluten-containing foods and *did not replace them with anything*, that person would probably lose weight due to a significant calorie deficit. But replacing gluten-containing foods with gluten-free foods actually can get us in trouble. Not only do these products typically contain fewer vitamins and less protein and fiber than wheat-based counterparts, but they also are usually higher in fat and sugar to improve the flavor and texture. They also often don't taste as good. Of course, there are exceptions, especially with manufacturing developments in the past few years. However, if given the option between a slice of freshly baked focaccia and a slice of gluten-free bread, most people I know would agree that the focaccia is the preferable choice. Just as with other food substitutions, avoiding gluten can lead to binge eating. If following a gluten-free diet is leading you to *over*eat gluten-free foods because they are less satisfying, I encourage you to reconsider your motivation for following the diet.

In general, extreme diet approaches should be reserved for extreme cases, most of which would already be monitored by a physician. Don't get me wrong; I'm not saying that we ought not to be proactive with our health. But on an individual level, when medicine isn't already your day job, sifting through the internet abyss to find health answers can be completely overwhelming, adding far more stress than it's worth. Instead, as I counsel my patients, the best way to manage your health is by focusing on cultivating a positive relationship with your body, building a relationship with a trusted health care provider for individual questions and concerns, and otherwise avoiding too much involvement in the health and fitness world. Most of the information that's shared online isn't helpful anyway, and any relevant information you might be missing will be delivered to you far more effectively by your health care provider. Sometimes, less really is more.

CHAPTER ELEVEN

Final Thoughts

When I got married, it took a little while for me to fully realize how significantly my life had changed. Before saying "I do," I knew I wanted something *more* in terms of experiences and intimacy with my soon-to-be husband, but having never been married before, I knew I had a lot of learning to do. Standing at the altar, I was overjoyed, excited, and a little nervous about the things to come. After the ceremony? I was exhausted, but I generally didn't feel any different from how I always had. I was the same Alexandra, only with a whole lot of adventures and learning ahead.

The changes started slowly. First, a new piece of jewelry always on my finger, followed by a second ring with my "I do." Then my husband moved into our apartment, and we started figuring out our daily routine: Who will make the coffee in the morning? What time will we go to bed? Then I changed my name at the social security office and applied for a new driver's license. Signing the name MacKillop? Now *that* felt weird! After my trip to the DMV, I almost had a mini identity crisis realizing that all my old habits were being challenged, and it was time to build something completely new. While I was thrilled to be a wife, I hadn't realized how much my behaviors had been centered on life as a single woman. Most of the changes were small, and I had anticipated them, but they still took getting used to—cooking twice as much food, discussing the nuances of our schedules in more detail, and the sweet experience of driving home together from Bible study in the evenings. But additionally, there were subconscious habits, like sleep talking and trying not to inadvertently steal all the blankets at night. My marriage affected every moment of my day, whether I was at home with my husband or not. While I did and still do love every aspect of being married, I was nonetheless surprised by the impact on my life of becoming united with another person.

The process of cultivating freedom in eating is very similar. Diet culture (and the pressure to look, eat, and exercise a certain way) touches every aspect of who we are, from our conversations, to our leisure activities, to our experiences at social events. Just as our families shape our behavior for the first decades of our lives, our eating patterns become deeply ingrained in the very flesh of our beings, even influencing our sense of identity. Therefore, just as with marriage, it's only reasonable to expect the process of cultivating a new relationship with food to be long, challenging, surprising, and emotional—and, of course, worth it.

Unlike a happy and healthy marriage, changing the way we approach food is also likely to be painful, stressful, and scary. Many of the rules we put in place for ourselves in terms of eating are there because we think they will keep us safe. We have been told all our lives that if we eat according to what our bodies tell us, we will completely lose control and suffer from the consequences. Diet culture makes us believe that our bodies are our enemies and that we need to override and subdue them to avoid becoming *fatter, uglier,* or *unlovable.* These lies are a far cry from the beauty that God spoke into his creation at the beginning of time. As you take each new step in this journey, cling to the truth that because you can trust God, the creator of all things, you can therefore also trust your body. God loves you and created you as an intentional expression of that love. As your body changes throughout your life, meditate on this knowledge. Even though this process of change may feel uncomfortable or unfamiliar to you, remember that you are known and deeply loved, and your body is doing exactly what it was made to do.

Persevering through the Ups and Downs

Over the course of my own intuitive eating journey, which I've been open and honest about in this book, I've had numerous ups and downs and shed many a tear. I even called it quits a couple of times, letting my guard down and dabbling in my old ways. But the discomfort and frustration of dieting always jolt me back to reality, reminding me why intuitive eating is necessary and good. When I allow thoughts about eating and exercise to cloud my heart and mind, I lose sight of what's important in my life—what truly fulfills me. The guilt, shame, and emptiness that accompany dieting bring me to my knees every time I stumble, and I end up shaking my head both in frustration and in resolve to live according to what is uplifting, right, and true.

In full disclosure, awareness of my own relapses contributed to my motivation to write this book. Beyond its purpose as a practical, guided health resource for readers, it serves as a personal manifesto. It's a way to remind my own heart of my tried-and-tested truth, alongside a collection of encouragements in times of struggle and an answer to the arguments that resurface when I relax my vigilance and let down my guard. Yes, I'm a doctor—an expert in the field—but I'm also human, and I'll be the first to admit that becoming an intuitive eater is anything but easy. In fact, it's probably one of the hardest things you'll ever do. Deciding to ditch dieting won't be a one-and-done type of ordeal. After a lifetime of food rules and body shaming, intuitive eating and self-acceptance feel like the least natural process ever. In the process, we literally rewire the neural circuits in our brains, and that is every bit as uncomfortable as it sounds. But with time, as you slowly cultivate awareness of your body's internal signals, experience the joy of food freedom, and understand how satisfying mindful eating can be, you'll establish your own sense of inner motivation to keep eating intuitively despite the discomfort. Once you've tasted and seen the goodness of God's original design for yourself, it'll be easier and easier to choose a life of fulfillment over restriction time and time again. Expect trials, tribulation, and temptation so that you can better equip yourself to overcome them.

Lasting Fulfillment

Dieting is like a math problem gone wrong. It tells us that if we subtract food, calories, energy, and freedom from our lives, we will be adding value. But it never works out that way. Weight loss won't make our lives better, and it certainly won't fulfill us. At the end of the day, our deepest need is to know that we are loved by the One who created us. As much as we may crave the approval of others (or even ourselves) for having a certain size body or eating a certain way, these things will ultimately never be able to deliver on their promises to us. Dieting for weight loss doesn't work, despite convincing claims to the contrary, as it ultimately creates more problems for us than it ever could have solved. From harming our health, to preoccupying our minds, to damaging our relationship with God and our bodies, depriving ourselves leads to disaster every time. But our alternative, intuitive eating, allows us to care for our bodies with kindness by honoring our health, responding appropriately to our needs, and reflecting God's love, which dwells within us. One of the most liberating truths of the gospel is that our bodies don't define who we are. In Christ, we are more than flesh and bone. We are more than what we look like, what we eat, or whether or not we face health struggles. As children of God, our identities are found in something so much bigger than a pants size, a serving size, or the number on the scale. These internal conflicts with dieting or with our weight grieve God perhaps even more than they concern us, for his desire is for each of us to fully know and understand the all-encompassing nature of his care and affection for us.

Life without God's love is empty. Without having our deepest need met, we turn to anything we can find that might promise to help us—things like dieting, losing weight, or otherwise attempting to change our bodies—and when those pursuits fail us, we have two choices: we can look for something else on this earth that may work a little better or last just a little bit longer, or we can come back to God, who is eternal. We can return to the design of our creator and commit to cultivating compassion and kindness toward our bodies as a reflection of his own. We can choose to love and care for ourselves as he loves and cares for us, living out his light in the world. Eating as God designed for us to eat, enjoying the satisfaction of nourishing food, and respecting the diversity of bodies he created, we can fully taste and see that he is good (Psalm 34:8); and not only is he good, but living in full awareness of his love is far better than dieting could ever promise to be.

Appendix

Here are some tips and tools designed just for you to use along your intuitive eating journey. Some of these tools might be more helpful for you than others. No need to use all of them! Just dive in and explore in whatever way you find the most helpful.

Food-Body Relationship Screening Tool

If you answer yes to any of the following questions, it may be an indication that you are struggling in your relationship with food and/or your body.

1 Do you find yourself distressed or depressed because of the size and shape of your body?

2 Does knowing your weight, pants size, or a sense of dissatisfaction with your appearance negatively impact your mood?

3 Do you struggle to notice positive qualities about yourself independent of your weight, shape, or size?

4 Do you find yourself repeatedly cycling through new dieting attempts without success?

5 Do you feel disconnected from your hunger and fullness cues and struggle to identify what and when to eat without an outside plan?

6 Do you feel compelled to exercise as a means of weight control rather than for enjoyment?

7 Do you believe that eating certain foods will harm your health and/or cause you to gain weight?

8 Do you make food choices based solely on nutrition/ingredients labels without paying attention to factors like taste, cravings, or satisfaction?

9 Do you feel guilty or ashamed for eating foods you enjoy?

10 Do you view food in black-and-white terms, such as good versus bad or healthy versus unhealthy?

11 Do you measure your food, count calories, or follow restrictions related to amount, frequency, or variety?

12 Do you feel distressed by your current approach to food?

13 Do you exercise to make up for episodes of overeating?

14 Do you feel you can't control yourself around certain foods, finding yourself overeating to the point of discomfort?

15 Do you struggle to maintain your weight, constantly cycling between weight gain and weight loss?

A Day in the Life of Intuitive Eating and Exercise

I share this as an example of what a day can look like, not as a prescription for how your foods and habits have to look. You'll eat different things at different times based on your own life and your own tastes. Enjoy the process of figuring out what this can look like for *you*.

A Day at Work

5:45 A.M. Wake up, get dressed, read the Bible, and prepare breakfast.

6:15 A.M. Eat breakfast: toasted Ezekiel bread with peanut butter and sliced banana and coffee with half-and-half.

7:00 A.M. Arrive at work and start my day.

9:00 A.M. Coworkers order takeout from a breakfast café. I'm still satisfied from breakfast and am not craving anything in particular. I choose not to place an order.

10:00 A.M. Eat a morning snack: cottage cheese and blueberries, plus a spare donut hole from the coworkers' breakfast order.

12:00 P.M. Eat lunch packed at home: pita chips, an orange, carrots with hummus, and leftover chicken fingers from a restaurant dinner the night before.

3:00 P.M. Exercise at the gym.

4:00 P.M. Arrive at home and eat two pieces of string cheese and a handful of grape tomatoes.

5:30 P.M. Shower, relax, and start making dinner.

6:15 P.M. Eat dinner: Thai curry with lentils, red peppers, cauliflower, and carrots served over white rice with dried mango and seltzer water on the side.

8:30 P.M. Eat dessert: mint chip ice cream with crushed Oreos.

10:00 P.M. Go to bed.

A Day at Home

9:30 A.M. Wake up, read the Bible, slowly start the day.

10:30 A.M. Eat a dried date with peanut butter as a snack while making breakfast.

11:00 A.M. Eat breakfast: coffee with half-and-half, boxed protein pancakes with butter, and sliced strawberries.

1:30 P.M. Eat lunch: leftover spaghetti squash with rotisserie chicken and melted cheese and a chocolate chip cookie. After the cookie, I'm not quite satisfied, so I eat another half of a cookie.

3:30 P.M.   Walk with my husband through the neighborhood.

4:30 P.M.   Eat a snack: iced coffee with half-and-half and a piece of banana bread with butter.

6:30 P.M.   Eat dinner: meatloaf with sweet potatoes, sautéed green beans, and a side salad with ranch dressing.

8:30 P.M.   Enjoy popcorn and a movie with my husband.

11:00 P.M.   Go to bed.

Structuring Your Food Framework

Each time you eat, strive to include a food from each nutrient category (protein, carbohydrate, fat, and fiber [fruit or vegetables]) at meals and from at least two at each snack. Rate your hunger/fullness before and after eating.

Meal	Nutrients	Hunger level before	Hunger level after
Breakfast	Protein: Carbohydrate: Fat: Fiber:	0–10	0–10
Morning snack	#1: #2:	0–10	0–10
Lunch	Protein: Carbohydrate: Fat: Fiber:	0–10	0–10

Meal	Nutrients	Hunger level before	Hunger level after
Afternoon snack	#1: #2:	0–10	0–10
Dinner	Protein: Carbohydrate: Fat: Fiber:	0–10	0–10
Dessert/snack		0–10	0–10

Discerning Your Motivation: Freedom versus Guilt

The following chart is another tool you can use to remind yourself of God's truth and help keep yourself accountable. The table outlines the principles discussed in this book, especially the contrast between actions motivated by guilt and shame versus actions motivated by love and freedom. All of these actionable steps are rooted in scripture, and the Bible reference is provided for each one as well. I encourage you to post this chart in areas where you can see it regularly. Write out the Bible verses on sticky notes and put them front and center in your home, in your car, or at your desk. The more we remind ourselves of the truth about God's love for us, the more likely we are to act on those truths.

Actions motivated by guilt and shame	Actions motivated by love and freedom	Scriptural reference
Avoiding dessert due to fear of weight gain	Enjoying your favorite foods, satisfying your cravings, and moving on with life	"So whether you eat or drink or whatever you do, do it all for the glory of God." (1 Corinthians 10:31)

Actions motivated by guilt and shame	Actions motivated by love and freedom	Scriptural reference
Reading diet and fitness theories or magazines	Reading devotionals that affirm God's love for you	"Keep this Book of the Law always on your lips; meditate on it day and night, so that you may be careful to do everything written in it. Then you will be prosperous and successful." (Joshua 1:8)
Following fitness models or "thinspiration" on Instagram	Unfollowing social media users who encourage unhealthy or extreme behavior	"If your right eye causes you to stumble, gouge it out and throw it away. It is better for you to lose one part of your body than for your whole body to be thrown into hell." (Matthew 5:29)
Reading and believing radical dieting statements online or in advertisements	Challenging the folly of dieting efforts and denouncing advertisements that encourage you to diet	"Do not conform to the pattern of this world, but be transformed by the renewing of your mind. Then you will be able to test and approve what God's will is—his good, pleasing and perfect will." (Romans 12:2)
Repeatedly checking your appearance (or shape) in the mirror	Covering large mirrors, choosing only to assess your appearance upon getting dressed	"Do nothing from rivalry or conceit." (Philippians 2:3a ESV)
Forcing your body into old clothes that are too small or buying clothes that you wish you could fit into but don't	Buying clothes that fit your "here-and-now" body and complement your unique shape and size	"For you formed my inward parts; you knitted me together in my mother's womb. I praise you, for I am fearfully and wonderfully made." (Psalm 139:13–14 ESV)

Actions motivated by guilt and shame	Actions motivated by love and freedom	Scriptural reference
Exercising to compensate for food indulgences	Exercising to relieve stress, strengthen your body, and feel energized	"For while bodily training is of some value, godliness is of value in every way, as it holds promise for the present life and also for the life to come." (1 Timothy 4:8 ESV)
Skipping meals to accommodate treats	Eating regular, balanced meals and enjoying treats too	"Go, eat your food with gladness, and drink your wine with a joyful heart, for God has already approved what you do." (Ecclesiastes 9:7)
Waking up too early to exercise	Sleeping enough because rest is more important than distance, calories, or the number on the scale	"'Come away by yourselves to a desolate place and rest a while.' For many were coming and going, and they had no leisure even to eat." (Mark 6:31 ESV)
Scrutinizing photos of yourself	Removing from view any pictures that spur self-deprecating thoughts	"Therefore encourage one another and build one another up, just as you are doing." (1 Thessalonians 5:11 ESV)
Neglecting your body because you don't like how it looks	Taking extra steps to do nice things for your body, like taking baths, washing your face, keeping your nails nice, or getting an occasional massage	"Be kind to one another, tenderhearted, forgiving one another, as God in Christ forgave you." (Ephesians 4:32 ESV)

Actions motivated by guilt and shame	Actions motivated by love and freedom	Scriptural reference
Engaging in all-or-nothing thinking with food ("I ate one cookie; I might as well eat the whole box.")	Engaging in satisfaction-motivated eating ("A cookie sounds good, so I'll eat one today. I will eat another one tomorrow if I want more. I can have cookies whenever I want.")	"If you find honey, eat just enough—too much of it, and you will vomit." (Proverbs 25:16)
Looking at nutrition labels to track calories, sugar, fat, etc.	Choosing foods that aren't served with nutrition labels	"Trust in the Lord with all your heart, and do not lean on your own understanding." (Proverbs 3:5 ESV)
Limiting or measuring food	Eating according to hunger and satisfaction	"For no one ever hated his own flesh, but nourishes and cherishes it, just as Christ does the church, because we are members of his body." (Ephesians 5:29–30 ESV)
Weighing yourself daily	Reducing weighing to once per week or month or throwing away the scale altogether	"For God gave us a spirit not of fear, but of power and love and self-control." (2 Timothy 1:7 ESV)
Buying diet products (or *reduced* products)	Eating full-fat, full-sugar, regular, original versions of your favorite foods	"God saw all that he had made, and it was very good." (Genesis 1:31)

Actions motivated by guilt and shame	Actions motivated by love and freedom	Scriptural reference
Wishing your body looked different	Focusing on things you are grateful for about the body you *have*	"Do not be anxious about anything, but in everything by prayer and supplication with thanksgiving let your requests be made known to God." (Philippians 4:6 ESV)
Comparing your body to others	Praising God for the diversity of his creation	"A tranquil heart gives life to the flesh, but envy makes the bones rot." (Proverbs 14:30 ESV)

Notes

Chapter 2

1. Deborah L. Jacobs, "For Working Women, Focus on Beauty Erodes Self Confidence," *Forbes*, April 23, 2014, https://tinyurl.com/y5jc328v.

2. Evelyn Tribole and Elyse Resch, *Intuitive Eating: A Recovery Book for the Chronic Dieter; Rediscover the Pleasures of Eating and Rebuild Your Body Image* (n.p.: Diane, 1995).

3. Tribole and Resch.

4. M. Hadjivassiliou, R. A. Grünewald, and G. A. B. Davies-Jones, "Gluten Sensitivity as a Neurological Illness," *Journal of Neurology, Neurosurgery and Psychiatry* 72 (2002): 560–63, https://jnnp.bmj.com/content/72/5/560.full.

5. Alan Levinovitz, *The Gluten Lie: And Other Myths about What You Eat* (Sydney: Read How You Want, 2015).

6. Steven Bratman, "What Is Orthorexia?," Orthorexia, 2014, http://www .orthorexia.com/what-is-orthorexia.

Chapter 3

1. Evelyn Tribole, *Intuitive Eating: A Recovery Book for the Chronic Dieter, Rediscover the Pleasures of Eating and Rebuild Your Body Image* (n.p.: Diane, 1995).

2. Tribole.

3. J. Obert, M. Pearlman, L. Obert et al., "Popular Weight Loss Strategies: A Review of Four Weight Loss Techniques," *Current Gastroenterology Reports* 19, no. 61 (2017), https://doi.org/10.1007/s11894-017-0603-8.

4. L. Lissner, P. M. Odell, R. B. D'Agostino, J. Stokes, B. E. Kreger, A. J. Belanger, K. D. Brownell, "Variability of body weight and health

outcomes in the Framingham population." *N Engl J Med.* 1991, 324: 1839–1844. 10.1056/NEJM199106293242602.

5. "Infertility Is a Global Public Health Issue," World Health Organization, June 28, 2019, https://tinyurl.com/y8kpylj2.

6. T. Mann, A. J. Tomiyama, E. Westling, A. M. Lew, B. Samuels and J. Chatman, "Medicare's Search for Effective Obesity Treatments: Diets Are Not the Answer," *American Psychologist* 62, no. 3 (2007): 220–33, https://www.ncbi.nlm.nih.gov/pubmed/17469900.

7. K. Strohacker, K. C. Carpenter, and B. K. McFarlin, "Consequences of Weight Cycling: An Increase in Disease Risk?," *International Journal of Exercise Science* 2, no. 3 (2009): 191–201, https://tinyurl.com/y263xj7b.

8. Obert et al., "Popular Weight Loss Strategies."

9. Bacon and Aphramor, "Weight Science."

10. D. Neumark-Sztainer, "Preventing Obesity and Eating Disorders in Adolescents: What Can Health Care Providers Do?," *Journal of Adolescent Health* 44, no. 3 (2009): 206–13, https://tinyurl.com/y5xdl57t.

11. Mayfield, "Whole as Whole Can Be."

Chapter 4

1. A. Smith, A. Baum, and R. Wing, "Stress and Weight Gain in Parents of Cancer Patients," *International Journal of Obesity* 29 (2005): 244–50, https://doi.org/10.1038/sj.ijo.0802835.

2. R. Rosmond, M. F. Dallman, and P. Björntorp, "Stress-Related Cortisol Secretion in Men: Relationships with Abdominal Obesity and Endocrine, Metabolic and Hemodynamic Abnormalities," *Journal of Clinical Endocrinology and Metabolism* 83 (1998): 1853–59.

3. "How Is BMI Used?" CDC, 2019, https://tinyurl.com/yy26g7sk.

4. Susan C. Wooley and David M. Garner, "Dietary Treatments for Obesity Are Ineffective," *British Medical Journal* 309 (September 10, 1994): 655–66, https://tinyurl.com/y279qjqn.

5. Michael Pollan, *In Defense of Food: An Eater's Manifesto* (New York: Penguin, 2008).

6. Jeanne H. Freeland-Graves et al., "Position of Nutrition and Dietetics: Total Diet Approach to Healthy Eating," *Journal of the Academy of Nutrition and Dietetics* 113, no. 2 (February 1, 2013): 307–17.

7. P. Rada, N. M. Avena, and B. G. Hoebel, "Daily Bingeing on Sugar Repeatedly Releases Dopamine in the Accumbens Shell," *Neuroscience* 134, no. 3 (2005): 737–44.

8. M. L. Westwater, P. C. Fletcher, and H. Ziauddeen, "Sugar Addiction: The State of the Science," *European Journal of Nutrition* 55 (Suppl. 2; 2016): 55–69, https://doi.org/10.1007/s00394-016-1229-6.

9. C. J. Lavie et al., "Exercise and the Cardiovascular System: Clinical Science and Cardiovascular Outcomes," *Circulation Research* 117(2) (2015): 207–19, https://doi.org/10.1161/CIRCRESAHA.117.305205.

10. Freeland-Graves et al., "Position of Nutrition and Dietetics."

11. Linda Bacon and Lucy Aphramor, "Weight Science: Evaluating the Evidence for a Paradigm Shift," *Nutrition Journal* 10, no. 9 (2011), https://tinyurl.com/ybj8bzyj.

Chapter 5

1. Jeremy M. Berg, "Each Organ Has a Unique Metabolic Profile," *Biochemistry*, 5th ed. (New York: US National Library of Medicine, 1970), section 30.2, https://www.ncbi.nlm.nih.gov/books/NBK22436.

2. Berg.

3. Berg.

4. Sally P. Stabler and Robert H. Allen, "Vitamin B12 Deficiency as a Worldwide Problem," *Annual Review of Nutrition* 24, no. 1 (2004): 299–326, doi:10.1146/annurev.nutr.24.012003.132440.

Chapter 7

1. Evelyn Tribole and Elyse Resch, *Intuitive Eating Workbook: Ten Principles for Nourishing a Healthy Relationship with Food*, A New Harbinger Self-Help Workbook (Oakland, CA: New Harbinger, 2017).

2. Barbara Gordon, "Eating Right Isn't Complicated," *Academy of Nutrition and Dietetics*, January 7, 2018, https://tinyurl.com/u7ctqfv.

Chapter 8

1. "Choose My Plate," US Department of Agriculture, 2019, accessed July 20, 2020, https://www.choosemyplate.gov/WhatIsMyPlate.

Chapter 10

1. K. Mitchell, "5 Thoughts," *Imma Eat That* (blog), September 3, 2018, https://immaeatthat.com/2018/09/03/5-thoughts-15.

2. K. Mitchell, "A Note about 'Healthy' Living Bloggers," *Imma Eat That* (blog), November 30, 2016, https://tinyurl.com/y248m5mh.

3. Ellyn Satter, "Take Good Care of Yourself with Eating," Ellyn Satter Institute, accessed July 14, 2020, https://tinyurl.com/ydj7tyog.